10⁰⁰

TWENTY YEARS OF COMMUNITY MEDICINE

A Hunterdon Medical Center Symposium

•

TWENTY YEARS OF COMMUNITY MEDICINE

A Hunterdon Medical Center Symposium

HIRAM B. CURRY, M.D.
ROBERT R. HENDERSON, M.D.
FREDERICK J. KNOCKE, M.D.
RICHARD M. MAGRAW, M.D.
JOHN SCHOFF MILLIS
EDMUND D. PELLEGRINO, M.D.
ANNE RAMSAY SOMERS
RAY E. TRUSSELL, M.D.
LLOYD B. WESCOTT
SAMUEL WOLFE, M.D.

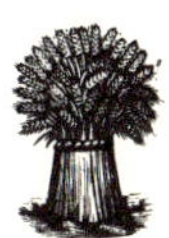

COLUMBIA PUBLISHING COMPANY, INC.
Frenchtown, New Jersey

*To the people of
Hunterdon County.*

●

CONTENTS

FOREWORD

In 1928 the Committee on the Costs of Medical Care* appointed by President Hoover reported the following:

> The Committee recommends that medical service, both preventive and therapeutic, should be furnished largely by organized groups of physicians, dentists, nurses, pharmacists, and other associated personnel. Such groups should be organized, preferably around a hospital, for rendering complete home, office, and hospital care. The form of organization should encourage the maintenance of high standards and the development or preservation of a personal relation between patient and physician.
>
> The Committee recommends that the costs of medical care be placed on a group payment basis, through the use of insurance, through the use of taxation, or through the use of both these methods. This is not meant to preclude the continuation of medical service provided on an individual fee basis for those who prefer the present method. Cash benefits, i.e., compensation for wage-loss due to illness, if and when provided, should be separate and distinct from medical services.
>
> The Committee recommends that the study, evalua-

---

* *Medical Care for the American People: The Final Report of the Committee on the Costs of Medical Care.* Adopted October 1, 1932. Chicago: University of Chicago Press, 1932.

tion, and coordination of medical service be considered important functions for every state and local community, that agencies be formed to exercise these functions, and that the coordination of rural with urban services receive special attention.

The Committee makes the following recommendations in the field of professional education: (A) That the training of physicians give increasing emphasis to the teaching of health and the prevention of disease; that more effective efforts be made to provide trained health officers; that the social aspects of medical practice be given greater attention . . .

Obviously, the time for these ideas was a long time in coming. Obviously, too, when a group of citizens in rural Hunterdon County, New Jersey, decided to build a medical facility in 1949, none of them was likely to have heard of the committee or its report. But what these citizens were ultimately to achieve in Hunterdon satisfied the committee's recommendations to a remarkable degree.

Hunterdon Medical Center opened its doors in the summer of 1953, the only hospital in a community of 40,000 people. A 100-bed institution, located in the middle of 45 acres of what was once cow pasture, it aspired to become a medical center providing a broad spectrum of services to an entire community.

In the ensuing 20 years, the center has grown along with the community. Hunterdon County's population more than doubled during this period; commercial activity increased substantially. Country roads have given way to interstate highways. One-room schoolhouses have disappeared. Huge regional educational facilities are now the rule. Vast shopping malls have replaced thousands of acres of farmland.

Despite this growth, and the ever-changing climate affecting medical care delivery, Hunterdon Medical Center has held to its convictions and, to a great extent, has achieved its goals.

To celebrate its 20th anniversary, Hunterdon and Princeton University sponsored a symposium at the university's Woodrow Wilson School on October 6, 1973. A grant from the Commonwealth Fund underwrote the cost.

Published here are the papers presented at the symposium. Five individuals, who were most closely associated with the development of the center since its inception, told how it started, how it responded to challenges, how it coped with problems, what its failures have been and to what extent it has succeeded in its mission—the first part of this book.

The first of them is Lloyd B. Wescott, a member of the original 1949 Board of Trustees who became president of the center in 1950 and continues in that capacity to this day.

The four speakers who followed were the first Medical Director of Hunterdon, Dr. Ray E. Trussell (1950-1955), and the men who succeeded him in that capacity: Dr. Edmund D. Pellegrino (1955-1958); Dr. Robert R. Henderson (1959–1970); and Dr. Frederick J. Knocke (1971 to date). Their narrative offers a continuing view of the operation of the medical center from the days before it opened until the present time.

Next, four nationally-recognized authorities discussed the four basic assumptions upon which Hunterdon functioned since its inception. They were asked to participate in the seminar not only because of their admitted expertise in the field of medical care delivery, but also because each had an early acquaintance with the medical center and its objectives.

The first speaker, Dr. Hiram B. Curry, is Director of the Family Practice Residency Program at Medical University Hospital, Charleston, South Carolina. He was followed by Dr. Samuel Wolfe, Director of Community Medicine for Long Island Jewish-Hillside Medical Center, New Hyde Park, New York. Next was Dr. Richard M. Magraw, President of the Norfolk, Virginia, Area Medical Center Authority. The final speaker was Anne Ramsay Somers, Associate Professor, Department of Community Medicine, New Jersey College of

Medicine and Dentistry-Rutgers Medical School and Research Associate, Industrial Relations Section, Princeton University.

Stated briefly, the four basic Hunterdon assumptions with which these authorities dealt during the symposium were:

• That the family physician would be an essential element of the health care system with a clearly defined role.

• That the family physician would be backed up by a closed, full-time, salaried, hospital-based staff of specialists.

• That a medical school affiliation and an active involvement in teaching was vitally important to insure the highest quality of medical care.

• That the community hospital should assume responsibility for, and serve as a focus for, the provision of a wide spectrum of health care services.

When Hunterdon opened, its affiliation with New York University Medical School was of enormous value. Through it, interns and residents were attracted on rotation from other affiliated New York hospitals. Hunterdon's specialist staff was able to profit from the stimulation and continuing education that a medical school affiliation affords. Above all, its greatest benefit was that it helped attract a specialist staff which included doctors of great distinction. To name but a few: Dr. Ray E. Trussell, now head of the Beth Israel Medical Center in New York; Dr. Edmund D. Pellegrino, formerly Director, Health Sciences Center, State University of New York at Stony Brook; and Dr. Andrew Hunt, now Dean of the Michigan State Medical School.

At another event in connection with Hunterdon's 20th anniversary, Dr. John Schoff Millis, a nationally recognized figure in the field of medical education, opened a panel discussion on the subject of the challenges which lay ahead. Because he identifies with such clarity a major problem facing not only Hunterdon but the nation as a whole in relation to the cost of medical care, we have included his provocative remarks herein.

We hope those of you who read this book will find it not only pleasurable but useful. It tells the story of a remarkable community effort involving many thousands of people who successfully developed a medical center based on concepts which now seem widely accepted.

We, the board of trustees, feel that the medical center has made great progress in fulfilling its commitment to the people of Hunterdon County. Year by year it has broadened the range of services provided. It has firmly resisted becoming what our president calls "a poor man's Mayo Clinic." The center has held firmly to its original aim to be the best community hospital possible for the people of Hunterdon. This has meant providing not only primary and secondary levels of care with ready and continuing access to tertiary care, but above all, reaching out beyond the walls of the hospital into the community and the homes of the people of Hunterdon. Many things remain to be accomplished. Many challenges lie ahead. We welcome them.

The Board of Trustees
Hunterdon Medical Center
Flemington, New Jersey

TWENTY
YEARS
OF
COMMUNITY
MEDICINE

A Hunterdon Medical Center Symposium

•

PART I

•

Hunterdon Medical Center
1953–1973

•

HUNTERDON MEDICAL CENTER: ITS BEGINNINGS

Lloyd B. Wescott

Since the Hunterdon Medical Center opened in July of 1953, it has attracted a surprising amount of attention in medical circles both in this country and abroad. In 1953, the institution seemed more innovative and unusual than it does now, but even today it appears to be doing some things that other institutions talk about doing. This, our 20th anniversary, seemed to be an appropriate time to look at what has happened here and think about what lies ahead for us. Hence, this symposium.

A few of us closely associated with Hunterdon will describe how it started, what the major influences affecting its development were, how it responded to these influences, and what its major successes and failures seem to have been.

Five distinguished authorities will discuss the underlying assumptions upon which Hunterdon has functioned, evaluating their importance, validity, and future applicability.

I, as chairman of the original study committee (1946) and director of the first fund drive (1949), will review the earliest years prior to the arrival, three years before the center opened, of our first medical director, Dr. Ray E. Trussell.

In discussing Hunterdon, it must be pointed out that, fundamentally, it is a voluntary community hospital. It receives minimal government support for charitable care. It has no endowment for operating deficits. As there is very little industry in the county, corporate support has been minimal. The families of Hunterdon built their medical center; they support it.

However, Hunterdon is more than the traditional community hospital. It is essentially an ongoing experiment in the delivery of high quality health care to a widely dispersed population. I say ongoing because while basic assumptions have not changed, the details of their application have responded to community growth and changes in the concepts of medical care over the years.

Much of Hunterdon's early history was told by Dr. Ray E. Trussell in his book.* I can—and sometimes do—talk at length about how Hunterdon started. Let me, however, give a few significant developments.

It is probably true that every unique institution is the result of a combination of time, place, and people. This is very true of Hunterdon.

As to time, the institution had its genesis in the meeting of the Hunterdon County Board of Agriculture in January 1946, when two concerned, local women, Mrs. Louise Leicester and Mrs. Rose Angell, came before the board to point out the county's acute need for improved medical services. World War II had ended. During that time the facilities of neighboring hospitals were gravely over-taxed and all too frequently it was impossible for us to find a hospital bed anywhere for our people. The need was apparent. These women urged the County Board of Agriculture to sponsor the construction of a hospital in the county.

As to the place, Hunterdon County lies equidistant between New York City and Philadelphia. It is a big county, 435 square miles. Incidentally, this is roughly the size of the four boroughs of New York City excluding Staten Island. The population at that time was around 40,000 people. The largest town, Flemington, the county seat, had a population of about 5,000.

In 1947, the economy of the county was essentially agri-

* Ray E. Trussell, M.D., *Hunterdon Medical Center: The Story of One Approach to Rural Medical Care.* Cambridge, Mass.: Harvard University Press, 1956.

cultural. It was one of the leading counties in the nation in the value of poultry and eggs produced and it was a significant factor in the dairy industry.

Hunterdon was the only county in the state without a hospital. About 20 active general practitioners provided the medical care for our dispersed population. Only five of them had formal hospital affiliations. None had training in a specialty.

The 40,000 citizens of Hunterdon County were and continue to be a remarkable group, conservative in some ways but self-sufficient and proud of their ability to provide for themselves. Over 500 of these citizens played active roles in the early fund drives. Of course, there were a few who played essential roles from the beginning.

Just a word about the County Board of Agriculture. It is a quasi-official, county-wide body of some 25 farm leaders, plus representatives of local industries, banks, schools, the clergy, the bar, etc. It has had an outstanding record of accomplishment over the years including the establishment of the first cooperative artificial breeding program for farm animals in the nation. Its president, Clifford Snyder, who later became the first president of the medical center, was a farmer of exceptional strength and distinction—a born leader.

The first response of the agriculture board to the proposal was negative. It was felt that no one wanted just another inadequate rural hospital and that to provide a first-class institution obviously was beyond our means. We agreed, however, that because of the need, the idea had to be explored and the study committee was appointed.

During that first year's planning we visited other hospitals in the state, received significant help from the New Jersey Department of Health and Hill-Burton* authorities and sought advice wherever we could find it. We were most strongly influenced by Dr. Lester Evans, then of the Com-

* A Federal program providing matching grants to build community hospitals where none existed previously.

monwealth Fund. Although he assured us that the fund had shifted its financial support away from hospitals and that we could not expect any grants, we repeatedly turned to him for advice. He is a most wise and reassuring man with a wealth of experience. Certainly he, more than any other, guided us in those early days.

After some months of study, the committee confirmed what it first assumed—that the building of a small rural hospital would not solve the community's health needs. Having a minimal hospital building would not guarantee that doctors would come to staff it. But we recognized that the county had virtually no public health services, school health programs were grossly inadequate, there were no visiting nurse services, no psychiatric services. No clinics were available for special treatment. Our few rescue squads were dependent upon the emergency rooms of hospitals in neighboring counties which, all too frequently, were overwhelmed with their own problems. As the committee recognized how great were the needs and how complex were the solutions in the area of health care, it asked the County Board of Agriculture for funds to employ a consultant. It was our great fortune to find Dr. E. H. L. Corwin, then the Chairman of the Public Health Committee at the New York Academy of Medicine. During 1947, as his time permitted, he studied the county's needs, evaluated the potential of the community, and met with local doctors and community groups. In January 1948, he gave us his report.

To determine that a hospital was needed was not difficult. He did point out, however, that we lacked many other things beside a hospital and fully documented all the deficiencies we had felt existed. His proposal was a challenging one—that we build a combination hospital and health center and that we seek an affiliation with a medical school. The last paragraph of his report reads as follows:

To sum up, if Hunterdon County were to build just

another hospital, I would be lukewarm to the proposition, but if this hospital is projected in terms of a progressive institution with a university affiliation, a model of its kind, able to bring what is best in medicine to the residents of a rural area and has associated with it an active full-strength health center and a good follow-through social service, I would be most strongly for it.

It is interesting to note in passing that Dr. Corwin's report warned us that the cost of operating a 125-bed hospital might run as high as $400,000 a year and that our per diem costs might be as high as $11.25. Oh, for the good old days!

I stated before that time always plays an important part in any significant new development. It is important to recognize that, in 1947, there were three factors that must have strongly influenced Dr. Corwin's recommendation.

The Hill-Burton program was just getting underway and he felt that a matching grant for construction would be available to us.

Also, at that time the New York University Medical School under a Kellogg Foundation grant had inaugurated a regional hospital plan designed to extend to community hospitals in and around New York an affiliation to assist them in providing programs in continuing medical education for their staffs. This is described in the book *A Mission in Action* by Drs. de la Chapelle and Jensen*, published in 1964. The university expressed an interest in establishing a truly close affiliation with a rural medical center, such as was proposed for Hunterdon.

Equally significant was the fact that, in 1947, the Commonwealth Fund published *Medicine in the Changing Or-*

---

* Clarence E. de la Chapelle, M.D., and Frode Jensen, M.D., *A Mission in Action: The Story of the Regional Hospital Plan of New York University*. New York: New York University Press, 1964.

der: A Report of the New York Academy of Medicine. This report proposed a new organization of health-care delivery, including a new type of institution that combined a hospital and a health center. The latter, the health center, would provide the more traditional public health services and together with the hospital would assume responsibility for providing a broad spectrum of medical care for the community at large. Dr. Corwin had worked on the New York Academy of Medicine book and his recommendations to us were certainly influenced by this.

Dr. Corwin's report, instead of dampening everyone's enthusiasm, seemed to be welcomed as a challenge. In March 1948, the medical center was incorporated. The name we chose—Hunterdon Medical Center—represented two commitments. We set ourselves to carry out Dr. Corwin's recommendation to build more than the traditional hospital and we undertook to serve all of Hunterdon, not just the area surrounding the proposed center. These two commitments strongly affected our subsequent plans.

During 1948, there were months of feverish work, countless community meetings, negotiations to assure us of a Hill-Burton grant, efforts to spell out our relationship with New York University, and explorations as to our fund-raising potential.

It became apparent that the community could accept generalizations about what was meant by a "health center" and it could accept in principle the value of the medical school affiliation. It was essential, however, that we have the whole-hearted support of the local doctors. This was not easy to get. The county medical society had formally endorsed the Corwin report before it was made public. Some of the doctors had strongly supported it from the first. Dr. Raymond Germaine, then president of the county medical society, played an active role in planning and became one of the original incorporators. However, many of the other doctors were genuinely skeptical. It sounded too grandiose. A few felt that as the planners were "a bunch of farmers" the whole idea was patently absurd.

Actually, Dr. Corwin's 1948 report had presented no details as to staff organization. As planning progressed, it became increasingly necessary to spell out what role the local physicians would play and how they would relate to the proposed specialist staff.

In August of 1948, Dr. Corwin gave us a second, shorter report which spelled out in more detail his proposed medical staff organization.

The report recommended that the staff be appointed by the medical center board on nomination of New York University Medical School and that it would "consist in part of those associated with the medical school and in part by the general practitioners. The heads of several departments—medicine, surgery, pathology, radiology—would hold academic rank on the faculty of the college and teaching obligations would be primarily though not exclusively in the Hunterdon Medical Center." It was recommended that these specialists be salaried. The other specialties were to be filled, for the time being, by residents at the end of their training, rotated out from the university or from one of the other affiliated hospitals. As to the local medical profession, the report stated that "all members of the local medical profession in good standing who expressed willingness to serve on the staff of the hospital will be appointed to positions of different grades on the attending staff depending on their qualifications, experience, and readiness to give of their time to the institution."

Control of the medical programs would be placed in the medical board of nine members—four salaried specialists and four general practitioners with the ninth member being a representative of the medical school.

This was still not specific enough to allay the uneasiness of the community doctors. Just what privileges would they have? How would they relate to a specialist staff that would certainly increase in size? What would they be expected to contribute by way of services to the medical center?

In searching for answers, we visited two hospitals that had medical school affiliations and whose staffs were closed to all but the hospital-based specialists. Medical care in the area immediately surrounding these hospitals was of high quality. However, it seemed to us that because the family physicians in the outlying areas were virtually excluded from any participation in hospital activities, their patients probably received less good care than they might have, had the hospital been organized on more traditional lines.

We not only needed the support of the local physicians to get the hospital built, we felt that the community-based family physician was essential to serve our widely dispersed population in the future.

In solving this problem, Hunterdon made what might well have been its most innovative and revolutionary decision.

It was decided that family physicians should be able to admit and retain their patients on medicine, pediatrics, and do non-complicated obstetrics. Hunterdon County people would be seen by specialists, either as in-patients or out-patients, only on referral from their family physicians and referred back as soon as medically justified. Thus, a continuing relationship between the patient and the family physician would be actively fostered. To assure quality medical care, each patient would be a teaching patient and seen on rounds, thus giving final responsibility to the director of the service. In addition, this provided continuing education for the family physician.

It was agreed that because some doctors practiced in communities far from the center, the traditional requirements for clinic and emergency coverage would not be required in return for staff privileges.

At the time, this seemed to us laymen a simple and obvious solution to our problem. In retrospect, we recognize how profound were the implications. That it worked and continues to work is due to the fact that the specialists and family physicians wanted it to work. Particular credit should go to two of our first specialists—Dr. Edmund D. Pellegrino, head of internal medicine, and Dr. Andrew Hunt, head of pediatrics. It was on these two services that the interface between the two groups of doctors was most direct and fraught with the greatest potential for misunderstanding.

In any event, the thesis adopted removed any active resistance on the part of the community doctors and we felt that we could move ahead.

The fund drive opened in the spring of 1949. I would like to tell you something about it as it strongly influenced subsequent developments. We decided not to use professional fund-raising help. The drive was strictly a home-grown affair. Our only employees were three local women. It was a most extraordinary success. The treasurer reported at the January 1949 meeting, at which we set the date for opening the drive, that our bank balance was $237.70. Twelve months later, he could report gifts and pledges totaling $977,000 from 7,140 donors. Our biggest single gift remained our first gift—a $50,000 pledge from a local industry. Our second largest gift was our second gift received—a $25,000 gift from our one really wealthy resident. In 1950, we had less than 65 gifts of over $1,000 each. Some 70 percent of the families in the county had contributed. Fund raising, of course, continued through planning and construction. The cornerstone contains the names of 10,000 donors, a record of a remarkable community effort. It is reassuring to report that this kind of support continues.

As I said, the fund drive had an effect on subsequent developments. We now had an irrevocable commitment to serve the entire county. It also meant that the community believed that this was to be their hospital in every sense of the word. Another result of this broad community support was that it convinced the Commonwealth Fund that something quite remarkable was going on in Hunterdon and they offered us a grant to hire our first medical director to help our dream become reality.

I would like to point out the receipt, at about this time, of another foundation grant which was vital to us. It was presumed that the full-time staff would charge the going rate for care rendered and that in time they would become self-supporting. This obviously was not possible in the early years. The Kress Foundation gave us a grant of up to $150,000 over a five-year period—$50,000 in the first year, $40,000 in the second, and so forth to cover deficits in the specialists' salary account. We did not need all of the first or second year's grants and by the end of the third year, the group was self-supporting.

We did have one significant failure in those early days. To fully implement Dr. Corwin's proposal we needed a county-wide public health department. As New Jersey law provides that every municipality (there were more than 20 of them in the county) was its own health authority, establishing a county-wide department was extremely complex, requiring petitions and referendums. The tradition of home rule in New Jersey is deeply embedded and at that time, in a rural community, public health meant either that someone was going to tell you to move your milkhouse or your outdoor privy, so there was a certain amount of built-in resistance. It seems an interesting commentary on the nature of this community that while they were giving the medical center the financial support needed, we were defeated almost 3 to 1 on the public health department referendum.

Actually, we now have a county health department but many of the traditional health department services are being rendered by the medical center or by other community organizations.

We did sustain one other disappointment. During our earliest planning years Dr. Evans urged us to consider providing a program for pre-payment of complete medical care for the county and urged us to study the Puget Sound plan. We did not for two reasons. We did not see how we could include the poor and near poor and we felt we had a commitment to the entire community. Also, we felt we had problems enough at that moment. Later we tried it. Dr. Knocke will tell you about this.

Except for these two failures, we have had extraordinary good fortune and have continued to work toward the full realization of our early dreams. One of our major good fortunes was a succession of four outstanding directors. They will describe how the medical center grew from these eager, hopeful beginnings.

HUNTERDON IN BRIEF RETROSPECT

●

Ray E. Trussell, M.D.
(Medical Director, 1950–1955)

As one looks back 23 years to an arrival in Hunterdon County as the first director of the yet-to-be-built Hunterdon Medical Center, one can only have a certain amount of wonderment that it ever happened.

It is true that Hunterdon was portrayed as a new and exciting venture. Certainly the board of trustees had already established their role as innovators by bringing in a director who was admirably suited to the challenge having never run a hospital let alone having had a course in hospital administration. Clearly, some communities have greater risk-taking capacities than others.

On arrival in Flemington, I was confronted with a headquarters on the second floor of a frame building, an open field which was to be the site of the future medical center, no written functional or architectural program, and an enormous sense of urgency and great expectation.

Hunterdon's board had achieved a minor miracle in securing a Hill-Burton grant in the face of original state-wide planning proposals which would have divided Hunterdon County between two other districts. To match this grant, a remarkable effort had been made to raise funds for construction and pledges totaling approximately $1 million were in hand. Humorously, it turned out that these pledges were in non-legal form and not acceptable to the New Jersey Hill-Burton authorities. A massive volunteer effort subsequently was necessary to re-secure the pledges in an acceptable form.

Some degree of the latent anxiety and potential hostility of local physicians was manifest in my first greeting by a family practitioner who simply stated, as his first words, "If this thing doesn't go our way, we'll sink your ship." Today, this physician is one of the staunchest supporters of the medical center and deeply involved in its day-to-day activities.

I also had been warned that the state medical society was viewing the entire project with misgivings and was prepared to sandbag me on my arrival. This prediction proved to be true in one sense, because during the five years I was in New Jersey, the successive presidents of the state medical society placed me on eight different state society committees and made me chairman of one. In addition, the local medical society reached the epitome of the unexpected by electing the director of the Hunterdon Medical Center as its president during his fifth year in the county. My experiences with organized medicine in New Jersey in those years and since were, with very rare exception, on the highest level of professionalism.

The medical center had its origins in the County Board of Agriculture. Thus, the board of trustees of the medical center had a considerable overlap with the parent board. Rarely is it the privilege of any hospital administrator to work with such a committed and hard-working group of people who were so supportive of the sophisticated leadership whom they had elected because of their long years of productive community activity in other fields. Even the most skeptical physician could not deny the commitment and almost spiritual sense of leadership which came from this group as they faced up to what seemed to be the impossible problem of creating a medical center in a rural county. What a contrast with some of the unfortunate inner-city self-selected "community leaders" some of us deal with today who are so committed to destruction.

The New York University regional affiliation program, which has been alluded to before, had foundered on the

Korean War and other natural events in the medical world. No longer was New York University geared to the idea of a massive network of affiliations which it would staff. Since the Hunterdon project had been agreed to some three or four years before, it had long since been forgotten except by a few key individuals. My first meeting with a committee of the faculty of New York University was a professional disaster and nearly led to the culmination of the project before it got underway. Fortunately, the administrative leadership of the medical school took prompt action to rectify the lapse in memory and commitment, primarily through the appointment of Dr. Clarence E. de la Chapelle as the liaison between the school and the Hunterdon Medical Center. This was, without any question, one of the most important events in the history of Hunterdon. It was Dr. de la Chapelle who guided us through the recruitment of our directors and who aided us in establishing the house staff rotations that became so popular after the program was launched. His dedication and faithfulness are a hallmark of Hunterdon's fame.

Had the Korean War not erupted, Hunterdon would have had a reasonably comfortable financial time during its construction period. Unfortunately, during the year that it took to develop the plans and get the final paper work out of the way, construction costs soared 35 percent. A national metal shortage was declared and a special trip to Washington was necessary to secure the first assignment of critical metals made to any hospital in the country.

As bids were opened, they were far beyond the financial ability of the medical center and, again, the sturdy underlying strength in Hunterdon County evidenced itself. Not only did the contractor and architects work in harmony to reduce the costs of the project, but the community responded in kind with a commitment to additional fund raising that exceeded anybody's worst expectations of what it would take to build a medical center.

There were other strengths in the total situation. Few

communities have benefited from the sophistication of a consultant like Dr. Corwin and the advice of a Commonwealth Fund staff, particularly people such as Dr. Lester Evans, Miss Mildred Scoville, Dr. Harry Handley, and others.

The Corwin report set the stage for not only a multiplicity of methods of community involvement in providing necessary health services but also for a unique arrangement of relationships between fully-qualified specialists to be imported and local family practitioners already serving. The underlying assumption in the Corwin report, which was never spelled out explicitly prior to the promulgation of the by-laws of the medical center, was the basic thesis that the full-time specialists who would be directors of their various departments had the ultimate responsibility for the quality of the care provided to all patients by all physicians and the responsibility for assuming such care if the problem was beyond the ability of the family practitioner. In conversations with Dr. Corwin, prior to his death, he was in full agreement that this was the critical issue on which the future of the medical center depended.

The Commonwealth Fund not only provided seed money towards development of the center, but at the last minute, in a break with policy, made an emergency grant of $250,000 towards the construction crisis. This encouragement, without any question, was one of the energizing factors in helping the community to face up to its over-all construction cost problems. In addition, a demonstration mental health program was mounted with Commonwealth Fund money, which could not conceivably have been undertaken without their assistance. There has been some misconception, however, that the Commonwealth Fund supported basic operating expenses of the medical center—an assumption which was never true. Whatever Hunterdon has done, it has done on its own.

Another problem which was confronted was the relative lack of public understanding of the specifics of what the medical center was to be. Many months were spent appearing before local groups ranging in size from six to 400 to interpret the program of the medical center. It was not unusual to encounter from time to time confusion, even resentment, about the projected relationship between the family physicians and the new specialists and about the fact that the specialist staff would be fully salaried and selected jointly with the help of the New York University Medical School where each specialist would have a faculty appointment. A number of self-selected specialists attempted to settle in Hunterdon, stating that they would be family physicians until the medical center opened, at which time they would expect to be on the staff and to restrict their practices to their specialties. More than one angry confrontation over the refusal of the board of trustees to allow this erosion of the program to which they had committed themselves was painfully worked through.

With the help of the New York University leaders, an excellent group of professional personnel was recruited for Hunterdon from a wide range of backgrounds and institutions. This recruitment included not only the directors of the various medical departments, but also the director of nursing. When the medical center opened, construction was still being completed in the basement and every service was to operate on a shoestring. These individuals who had all come from large training centers with a multiplicity of personnel and services found themselves trying to perform miracles with such limited resources. The degree to which they succeeded is beyond all expectation.

I can remember discussions not only with local community representatives but with the Commonwealth Fund staff about their fear that having nine full-time specialists on hand on the day of the opening of the medical center was far too rich in staffing and that we could not afford it. At the present time, I understand there are more than 30 full-time specialists and the program is still expanding. However, in the early days everyone was spread very thin. Our then director of surgery, Dr. Carl Roessel, whose untimely death saddened us all, was on call 24 hours a day, seven days a week. The same kind of problem faced every director.

Our director of nursing, Miss Lela Greenwood, opened the hospital with barely enough nurses to get half of the beds underway. Ultimately, she brought together a nursing staff from more than 45 different schools of nursing and welded them into one cohesive unit whose performance evoked the admiration of physicians and community alike.

Since our director of medicine, Dr. Pellegrino, and our director of nursing were both Bellevue Hospital products, it is not surprising that I had a deep admiration for the Bellevue tradition long before I became New York City Commissioner of Hospitals and found Bellevue as one of my lesser headaches. At Hunterdon, I could hardly wait to get the morning report from Miss Greenwood to find out what had gone wrong and what she thought we should do about it. It was one of the finest on-the-job and face-saving courses in hospital administration any director could ever have. Dr. Pellegrino's performance not only in the center but in relation to the practicing profession in New Jersey and Pennsylvania was exemplary and had much to do with the widespread acceptance of the medical center within the first year. I could make similar comments about our other pioneers.

Of course, along with all of this we were conducting the chronic illness survey for the National Commission on Chronic Illness.* This was a massive enterprise which provided Hunterdon with more information about the health of its constituency than any other facility in the history of the world. It also was an enterprise which occupied an enormous amount of personnel time, community involvement, and the development of certain unique services such as multiple

---

* Ray E. Trussell, M.D., and Jack Elinson, M.D., *Chronic Illness in a Rural Area: The Hunterdon Study*. Cambridge, Mass.: Harvard University Press, 1959.

screening and extensive application of the diagnostic center services to a random sample of the county's population.

I would be remiss in writing a paper such as this after 20 years of operation of the medical center without paying tribute to the staff who were willing to join in the beginning in this unproven venture and to the strong support which we received from the New York University medical hierarchy. The local community was indeed fortunate to have the help; the professionals were indeed fortunate to have the community so supportive and understanding.

The Hunterdon Medical Center Board of Trustees has brought together and expanded the necessary resources to serve as the backbone of a health care resource which is reaching out to provide help locally where it is needed. We in the large city have had experiences with this in such situations as the Gouverneur Health Services Program on the Lower East Side of Manhattan staffed by Beth Israel Medical Center and the Judson Health Center in turn staffed by Gouverneur. The Martin Luther King Health Center staffed by Montefiore is a similar example.

Hunterdon, with its facility in Lambertville and its plans for similar facilities elsewhere, likewise can help fulfill the health services requirements of the community as they unfold.

In retrospect, as I look back at Hunterdon, among the many outstanding accomplishments the single most exceptional feature has been that of the use of medical personnel of different degrees of training, goals, and interests and their working relationships within the same community. There are, in the world, various patterns of medical organization. To mention a few—Hunterdon is the exact opposite of the British form of providing care between the combined efforts of the family practitioner, who is essentially outside of the hospital, and the specialist, who is inside. Hunterdon also differs from the Mary Imogene Bassett Hospital in Cooperstown, New York, by virtue of including community-based family practitioners whom Cooperstown as a matter of policy excludes. Hunterdon also differs from the Kaiser Foundation system where all physicians, both family practitioners and super-specialists, are on the payroll and part of one organization. As such, Hunterdon deserves to be placed in the array of organizational efforts in this country to achieve high-quality and locally-available medical care under voluntary auspices and to be evaluated on the same terms as other experiments which this nation has fostered. Hunterdon also is in a unique position to respond to almost any form of national health insurance which may evolve in the Congress, hopefully sooner rather than later. Certainly in terms of meeting the needs of a semi-rural population, Hunterdon has gone further than most.

TWO DECADES BEFORE ITS TIME

●

Edmund D. Pellegrino, M.D.
(Medical Director, 1955–1960)

The Hunterdon Medical Center—20 years after—is living proof against the common sense notion that ideas born before their time rarely survive. Of equal rarity is the opportunity we enjoy today for a 20-year follow-up of ideas born before their time. Almost all the principles upon which Hunterdon is built were hotly disputed two decades ago; some were considered merely impractical, others aberrant, and some downright heretical and sure to mean the end of quality medical care if they were allowed to persist. Even friendly observers thought us a bit foolhardy and were amazed that the brave attempt did not falter but actually succeeded in most of its aims.

Today, most of the ideas that constitute the Hunterdon plan are considered essential to proper community planning for comprehensive health services. Those ideas did not originate at Hunterdon. They had existed in disjointed form in a number of institutions. Hunterdon's great contribution was to take a group of relatively new ideas, implement them in one institution, and unite them around a common mission —to provide the highest possible care for the people of a rural community.

I want to limit myself to a few of these seminal ideas about health care, professional relationships, and the nature of community hospitals which have been explored at Hunterdon. Whether the clear identification of these principles now is more an act of retrospective rationalization than of prospective intuition can be debated. Some of my colleagues favor a more empirical interpretation of how these concepts grew. With the safeguard of geographic and chronologic distance, I wish to suggest that what is now the Hunterdon plan grew in a rational and analytic way out of the need to provide solutions to a series of health care problems which faced a rural county in 1953. These solutions admittedly took place within a very special matrix of commitments made by community leaders. They had opted for the most constructive, if not the safest, thinking they could bring to the situation. Rarely, in my experience, has the blend of community commitment and professional willingness to explore new avenues been so nearly in conjunction. And so effectively reinforced by cooperation with a major university.

In my memory still, from the time of my interview for the job of director of internal medicine, is the oft-repeated assertion by trustees that Hunterdon did not want an "ordinary" hospital. No one quite knew what the alternatives were, but they knew that above all they must not be ordinary —and indeed they have not been. That determination to meet problems in new ways was accompanied by the courage to persevere with new ideas long enough to probe their utility. It has often been said that Hunterdon was a unique institution. If there was something unique, it was this determination on the part of community leaders to support the creative efforts of a young, largely untried professional staff who came to Hunterdon because it promised not security or success but the chance to test their ideas. The subsequent careers of the original staff show they were a special breed who had selected Hunterdon as much as it had selected them.

Like Ray Trussell, I, too, was largely unqualified for the tasks I was to undertake. I was reasonably well trained in clinical internal medicine but completely unacquainted with community medicine, which is what we were practicing, though it had not yet been named. Like Ray, I, too, was also unqualified for running a hospital, which I did when he left for Columbia and I added the position of hospital director to my portfolio. With the kindness of the board, the patience of Lloyd Wescott and Seward Johnson, Dr. Clarence E. de la Chapelle, and the capable administrative support of Ed Grant, I eventually learned enough about hospital administration to avoid impeding their efforts.

Equally fortuitous were the courage and the foresight exhibited by the Commonwealth Fund which assisted in the support of this unique configuration of ideas and people. Even more important than fiscal support were the advice, support, cajoling, and stimulation so wisely and genially provided by Lester Evans, M.D., then executive associate of the foundation. Evans immediately grasped the special potentialities of Hunterdon and reassured all of us—staff, board, and practitioners—of the probity of our ideas whenever some crisis threatened to damage our resolve.

Let us look at a few of the practical problems we faced and the solutions that emerged. In the solutions, we shall find the seminal ideas of the Hunterdon plan, which have survived for 20 years and which are essential for other community hospitals seeking to meet the needs of the people they serve.

RELATIONSHIPS WITH THE PROFESSIONAL COMMUNITY

Prior to the opening of the hospital, the professional needs of Hunterdon County were being provided by between 20 and 30 active general practitioners. It was essential that their services should continue and be complemented and supplemented by the staff of full-time specialists who would confine their work to the hospital. Nothing would have been more deleterious to the medical care of the community or more fatal to the whole enterprise than friction or open rupture on the professional front. We all knew that for optimal care every community needs both family and general practitioners, as well as specialists. Very few examples existed of how these two groups could work synergistically. Indeed, there was an impressive record of failure elsewhere to sober us. If there was one rock on which the whole enterprise could founder, this was it!

The context within which these relationships were to be worked out was literally a mine field strewn with opportunities for detonation every few feet. The trustees had vested the responsibility for the quality of hospital care in a group of young specialists, all of whom had faculty appointments at a "distant" medical school in New York City, one with few alumni in that part of New Jersey. The practitioners had every right to be anxious about the impact of these inter-lopers upon their established modes of practice. Though the county medical society had agreed to cooperate, this compact could be vitiated by one false step, however well-intentioned. That this did not happen then, or since, and that the relation-ships are still excellent, is a tribute to both the full-time specialists and the practitioners of the county. It also reflects the fact that the relationship had elements of enlightened self-interest built into it by both sides. Some of the details are of importance because of their applicability to other institutions and to problems of professional interrelationships which are yet to be resolved in either academic or practice settings.

All practitioners in good standing with the county society were automatically admitted to the attending staff of the hospital. All were general and family practitioners. The absence of specialists in the county removed one serious dimension of conflict. From time to time over the years, specialists did ask to join the staff, but the board held to the principle of a closed specialist staff. This is admittedly a debatable issue and it will certainly recur.

General practitioners were granted privileges in medicine, pediatrics, normal obstetrics, and minor but not major surgery*. They admitted patients directly to these services and

---

* Edmund D. Pellegrino, M.D., "Role of the Community Hospital in Continuing Education—The Hunterdon Experiment." *Journal of the American Medical Association*, 164(4):361–65, May 1957.

had three options with respect to the specialist staff. They could rely on the routine review of their cases by the chief of service as part of his daily rounds; they could ask for formal consultation with the specialist, retaining their role as attending physicians; or they could transfer the patient to the full-time staff, resuming his care upon discharge. Frequent informal consultation between attending general practitioners and the specialist staff was essential, especially in medicine and pediatrics, where the majority of patients were attended by the general practitioners. In obstetrics, normal deliveries were performed by the general practitioner, but complicated deliveries were the responsibility of the specialist staff.

The specialist staff did not charge fees for routine supervision, but it did charge in the case of either the formal consultation or taking charge of the full care of the patient. The most delicate relationship was the one in which the general practitioner remained the responsible attending physician, and the specialist saw his patient on daily rounds. The specialist had responsibility for the standards of care on the service and had to exert this responsibility in the most diplomatic fashion to avoid embarrassment to the attending general practitioner and confusion for the patient. Both wrote notes and orders on the chart and communicated with the house staff. The possibilities of conflict of opinions, overlap of authority, and unintentional lapses in communication were numerous.

Yet, in my six years at Hunterdon, only one case involving a sharp difference of opinion ever came to the medical board for adjudication. It concerned the need for gynecologic consultation. The board, consisting of equal numbers of specialists and general practitioners, voted to support the action of the full-time specialist.

Important elements in the professional relationships were the equal representation on the medical board of community practitioners and full-time specialists; a functioning professional staff organization that included all physicians, full-time staff and family practitioners; and effective communications between all physicians, the board, and the medical director. Family physicians were members of all hospital committees, taking part in teaching and all aspects of planning. Specialists, in turn, were active members of the county medical society.

Equally essential was the policy in the diagnostic center that specialists should see patients only on referral from a community physician. Patients were referred back to the physician promptly, usually with both a personal and a written consultation report. In the emergency room, patients were seen as they appeared, of course, but they were always asked to identify their family practitioner if they had one and wished him to be called. While patients without physician referral were seen whenever they insisted, the value of having a family physician in the community was always emphasized to them. Such patients were provided with lists of community physicians on the hospital staff who would provide continuing care.

The specialist staff, therefore, made a clear effort to function as consultants, assisting the community physician in hospital and ambulant care but not displacing him as the essential resource in primary medical care. The generalist in his turn recognized the utility of specialist attention in secondary and tertiary care. The family physician's role in hospital care was to provide those unique contributions that derive from his knowledge of the patient and the family and his interest in the pre- and post-hospital portions of the patient's medical life history.

The general practitioners thus became, from the outset, an integral part of the total health care system in the county. The responsibility for primary care was their most important mission. But they were also the integrating elements in the secondary and tertiary levels of care. The benefits to patients were clear. The community had the benefit of both specialist and family medical care; all levels of care were coordinated with each other and available in one community. The only exceptions were the most complicated problems which were sent to the university centers of New York or Philadelphia.

The relationship of the family practitioner with the specialist has proven itself over the last 20 years. It offers a model of how these relationships could be established in other institutions. One of the major deterrents to effective integration of family practice departments in medical schools and larger medical centers is the relationship between generalist and specialist in the care of the hospitalized patient. The Hunterdon experience offers a viable resolution for university as well as community medical centers*.

HUNTERDON AS A TEACHING HOSPITAL

The Corwin report asserted that Hunterdon should be associated with a university and participate in teaching, on the thesis that this association would tend to better patient care. Hunterdon's establishment was timely in this respect, since New York University was at that time committed to a regional affiliated hospital program in the metropolitan area.†

With the assistance of Dr. Clarence E. de la Chapelle** and Dr. W. N. Hubbard†† of New York University, fourth-year medical students were offered electives at Hunterdon and interns were rotated from St. Vincent's and Lenox Hill Hospitals in New York City.

Hunterdon had unique educational experiences to offer

* Edmund D. Pellegrino, M.D., "The Identity Crisis of an Ideal." In *Controversy in Internal Medicine II*. F. J. Ingelfinger, R. V. Ebert, M. Finland, and A. S. Relman, eds. Philadelphia: W. B. Saunders Co., 1974, in progress.
† Clarence E. de la Chapelle, M.D., and Frode Jensen, M.D., *op. cit.*
** Dr. de la Chapelle at that time was associate dean of the postgraduate medical school and Director of the Division of Regional and Affiliated Hospitals of New York University.
†† Dr. Hubbard at that time was associate dean of the medical school of New York University.

medical students and interns—something still unavailable to many medical students today. This was the opportunity to work with practicing family physicians, to learn about clinical medicine in a setting which served patients of all socioeconomic characteristics, to see health and illness in the context of a defined community experience, and to experience the possibilities inherent in comprehensive health services for a total community. This was community medicine long before the discipline was baptized and recognized as an entity of its own.

These pedagogic aims were achieved while each patient also had a responsible attending physician who was supervised by the full-time specialist staff. Students were thus enabled to see models of professional cooperation for the benefit of the patient. They appreciated that one standard of behavior could be, and indeed must be, exhibited whether one deals with the poor or the well-off. All patients, regardless of their ability to pay, were seen by students and house staff. Despite the private status of all patients, I can remember only one patient who refused to participate in the educational program. Even this patient eventually asked to be included.

Perhaps more importantly, the student could appreciate that physicians will find it difficult to cooperate with other health professionals unless they first learn to cooperate in a true team relationship with each other. The specialist-family physician team is the backbone of comprehensive medical care. We are still far from making the full spectrum of medical services available to all patients in an articulated way in most communities.

The only residency programs we attempted were in family medicine. Twenty years ago family medicine did not have the status it has achieved today. Indeed, most residencies went begging. Yet Hunterdon, because of the unique professional relationships it had undertaken, provided opportunities for educating the family physician of the future. Our residencies were filled for these reasons. But more significantly, the residents who trained at Hunterdon Medical Center also settled in Hunterdon County to practice. Over the years the reservoir of family physicians was replenished and then expanded. This was certainly not the experience of other rural communities during the same two decades.

Hunterdon, therefore, was an essential, unique, and effective learning experience for the students and staffs of several medical schools. The pedagogic objectives it set for itself and the experiences it provided were indeed ahead of the times. Only recently have they become common practice in many medical schools.

Perhaps the most significant educational effort was in the continuing education of family practitioners. This was made a part of their daily care of the practitioners' patients in the hospital and out-patient service. The full-time specialists constituted a cadre of *in situ* faculty who could be consulted informally on any problem, who conducted teaching rounds and seminars. They themselves were kept abreast of recent developments by their weekly visits to teach and learn as members of the faculty of the NYU Bellevue Medical Center.*

The focus of continuing education was the practitioner's own patient, thus capturing his motivation to help that patient by learning more about his problem and the way to resolve it. Every contact with the family physician was made a teaching occasion during the daily rounds by the full-time specialist staff, in the written and oral reports of an out-patient consultation, as well as in more formal rounds and seminars. The opportunity for continuing education was consciously made an intrinsic element in every facet of the family physician-specialist relationship.

As we enter the era of mandatory continuing education of all health professions, the methods and the experiences gained at Hunterdon are more than ever pertinent. With the

* Edmund D. Pellegrino, M.D., "Role of the Community Hospital in Continuing Education—The Hunterdon Experiment," *loc. cit.*

themes of quality assurance and accountability running through recent Federal legislation, it is clear that continuous, *in situ* continuing education is the only really effective method for a busy practitioner.

Hunterdon thus pioneered in medical education at all levels and in directions that have since come to be appreciated nationally as essential for most students and physicians. It did so with the full cooperation of patients, practicing physicians, and the community, all of whom perceived the benefits to be derived when teaching is truly an integrated part of patient care. This was accomplished without "turning over" the patient to the student or house staff or, on the other hand, limiting his participation in patient management.

COMMUNITY HOSPITAL OR COMPREHENSIVE COMMUNITY HEALTH CENTER

When community representatives said they did not want an "ordinary" hospital, they probably had little conception of how broad a spectrum of services was eventually to be offered. Hunterdon was surely one of the few community hospitals of its size to offer services that spanned curative, preventive, and rehabilitative medicine, coordinated in-patient and out-patient care, housed most of the voluntary health agencies in the county, and served as the focal point for all health services. I have borrowed a diagram from an earlier paper to summarize the breadth of services available (Figure 1).* This range of services is certainly not what one would have found in most hospitals 20 years ago, and it is still not available in most community hospitals today.

* Edmund D. Pellegrino, M.D., "The Role of the Local Community in the Development of Health Services—The Hunterdon Experiment." In *Industry and Tropical Health,* Vol. IV. Boston: Harvard School of Public Health, 1961.

FIGURE 1

INTEGRATION OF COMMUNITY HOSPITAL AND HEALTH CENTER FUNCTIONS HUNTERDON MEDICAL CENTER

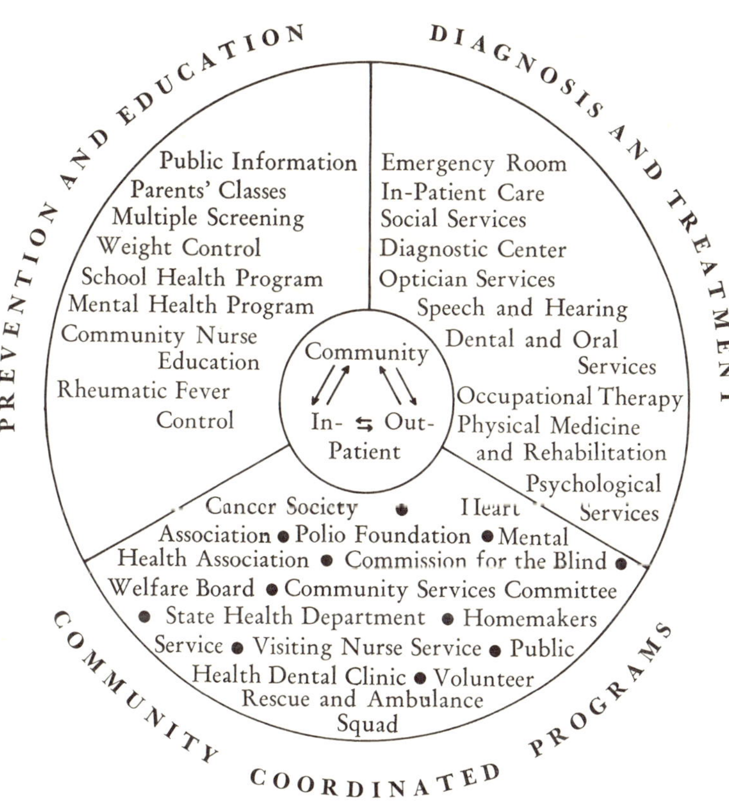

The community hospital commands the bulk of resources needed to meet the needs of the people it serves. It is distressing today to see hospitals bypassed for failure to appreciate the essentiality of their development as more comprehensive instruments encompassing all dimensions of patient and community care. The Hunterdon Medical Center was among the first to anticipate the direction of the evolution the community hospital must undergo to be truly responsive to all the health needs of the community it serves. (One of the reasons hospitals have not undertaken the central role they should play in planning for and providing comprehensive health services in the community is their failure to appreciate the need to become community health centers.)

In broadening the spectrum of its services, particularly in community psychiatry, patient education, preventive services, and rehabilitation, the trustees, staff, and community were not without their doubts. But Hunterdon's commitment to something more than the "ordinary" drew it inevitably to an exploration of the full extent of services a community requires.

COMMUNITY PARTICIPATION

One of the distinctive features of Hunterdon, which impresses all but the most casual visitors, is the sense that the hospital really *belongs* to the community. This cannot be quantitated or even evaluated in any clear way. Yet, from the outset, as my colleagues Mr. Wescott and Dr. Trussell have already indicated, the major impetus for the center came from the community, albeit through its informed leaders. This was attested in concrete terms in the initial and subsequent fund drives. Dollar contributions were more than matched by hours of volunteer services in every department. Much of the air of personal concern and humanity which pervaded the institution has come from encounters of patients and visitors with their neighbors serving in a hundred different capacities.

Every major planning effort, change of program, and evaluation of service evolved out of a continuing dialogue with the community. Despite some demurs from time to time, there was at Hunterdon more sense of community participation than I have experienced subsequently. This quality, subtle though it was, is in my mind a vital ingredient that enabled new and unproved programs to grow in that atmosphere of trust without which they can so easily be snuffed out. The confluence of community interest with that of the board of trustees, the professional staff, and the practicing physicians was remarkable. This confluence can hardly have been fortuitous, though I can describe its precise chemistry only vaguely.

FISCAL VIABILITY

Hunterdon as a private voluntary community hospital had to make its way in the world of fiscal realities despite its high commitments and courageous experiments. Dr. Trussell has pointed out how dubious in the minds of some was the acquisition of such a large staff of full-time specialists. Others worried about the wide span of services, especially those that were poorly remunerative, and about the amortization of what were considered to be large capital investments for a small community. The subsequent expansion of the center and its future plans are evidence enough that bold and new programs can be sustained out of community resources without extraordinary outside fiscal infusions.

There were deficits. Some in the early years were quite alarming. They were always balanced at year's end by substantial community participation in fund drives. There was general acceptance of the fact that deficits represented services needed by Hunterdon County residents who could not afford to pay for them, rather than poor management. This acceptance was based on that sense of participation to which I referred earlier.

SOME MISSED OPPORTUNITIES

Despite the evident success of the major features of the Hunterdon plan, there were some notable missed opportunities. Had these opportunities been seized, Hunterdon would now be even more effective as an instrument of community service than it is. I will mention two of these because of their current importance on the health care scene in this country: failure to establish public health and community medicine as a department in the center, and lack of development of a pre-payment insurance plan for the county, with the center as its base.

The reasons for not undertaking these programs are too complex to detain us now. In retrospect, their importance to a truly comprehensive program is more evident today than it was 20 years ago. Community medicine has become a discipline in many medical schools, and a number of community hospitals are beginning to make community medicine a full-fledged service, fully integrated, as it should be, with all other aspects of medical care. Pre-payment is so current a topic and of such broad interest that it needs no comment here. Suffice it to say that the Hunterdon plan offered almost unique possibilities for such an endeavor. Hunterdon might have exemplified the way smaller communities could move to pre-payment plans.

SOME STILL UNANSWERED QUESTIONS

Two questions have recurred over the years among the observers of the Hunterdon plan: How can its effects be evaluated? Why has such a successful plan not been reproduced elsewhere?

These are unlikely to be answered in any satisfactory way even now, least of all by those of us who were so intimately related to Hunterdon.

So far as evaluation goes, it is regrettable that we did not build in prospective methods of evaluation of the impact of the Hunterdon Medical Center in the health care of the community. The chronic illness survey* was supposed to be one such mechanism permitting serial comparisons of the impact of the center on the prevalence, incidence, morbidity, and mortality due to chronic illness, but adequate follow-up surveys using the same criteria as the original study are unlikely to be done. Such a study would probably not yield fully reliable information, since so many features of the epidemiology and ecology of chronic illness have changed in the intervening years. Moreover, it will be difficult to make comparisons, since the clinical observers will be different people with different criteria. Prospective studies of the impact of Hunterdon are still possible, but, like retrospective evaluation, they would lack adequate controls.

Process evaluation may be a little more promising than outcome analysis. This could be studied even if a control community could not be identified. Two possibilities suggest themselves:

(a) Evaluation of the effectiveness of Hunterdon in achieving the goals it set for itself 20 years ago and will set for itself in the future. This evaluation against an internal standard would have value for Hunterdon as well as for outside observers.

(b) The Hunterdon program could assess itself against some of the common objectives of any health care system—accessibility, availability, effectiveness, efficiency, patient and physician satis-

---

* Ray E. Trussell, M.D., and Jack Elinson, M.D., *op. cit.*

faction, and other factors. Here, a control community and hospital would have to be identified.

Important information for Hunterdon and other community
hospitals could eventuate from either approach.

FUTURE DIRECTIONS

There are many new directions Hunterdon might take. And,
despite its successes, Hunterdon like any living organism
must grow and develop or it will undergo senescence. I would
like to emphasize only one—preventive medicine.

The development of a plan for community-wide preventive medicine and health education will be an essential for
every hospital. This service is needed now to complement the
range of services Hunterdon already provides. Prevention is
always more admired in theory than practiced. Indeed, no nation or community has yet applied the knowledge we now
have of prevention for the benefit of all its members. Hunterdon Medical Center could do so admirably.

This is not the place to outline such a program in detail.
But the basis would be a vigorous application of what we
know about diet, exercise, smoking, accident prevention, and
emotional health as factors in mortality and morbidity of
some of our most important diseases. An individualized prescription of preventive measures for patients like the individualized prescription in curative medicine is needed. Reinforcement and follow-up for abnormalities in screening coupled
with personalized and group educational programs could
eventuate in a truly effective community-wide program of
health maintenance.

Why has Hunterdon not been replicated elsewhere? This
question has puzzled many. Was the confluence of favorable
circumstances, people, and ideas so unique as some have said?
Or are there identifiable factors inhibiting the development

in other communities? Unquestionably, Hunterdon enjoyed special advantages: a community without a hospital, without entrenched specialists, coupled with enlightened community leadership and university affiliation. These four factors in conjunction were indispensable to success. They are not often found in precisely this combination elsewhere.

I have had two personal experiences attempting to transplant the Hunterdon idea, once at Morehead, Kentucky, and again in a new institution in the Hamptons on Long Island. The first was only partially successful; the second is proceeding well but has yet to begin operation. I am certain there will be others.

Ideas born before their time can indeed survive, but they require a special nutrient medium. Hunterdon provided that medium 20 years ago. I believe the next two decades will see many more replications, because those ideas that were strange and out of their time then are now becoming evident needs in many communities. Yesterday's heresies often become today's orthodoxies in health as in theology.

What hospital boards and staffs have not done, community pressures will bring about because the elements of the Hunterdon plan are fundamental to any comprehensive community health care system. It is Hunterdon's special accomplishment that these ideas could be tested there before their time. Their success should embolden community hospitals elsewhere to become community health and teaching centers with alacrity and enthusiasm and before external events impose these patterns from without.

Twenty years later Hunterdon is still a viable, successful model community hospital. Hopefully, the courage to be different which the people of Hunterdon exhibited will inspire like courage in other communities.

HUNTERDON DURING A CHANGING ERA

•

Robert R. Henderson, M.D.
(Medical Director, 1960–1970)

I arrived at Hunterdon the week before the center opened and spent the next 17 years as a fellow, a member of the department of internal medicine, director of that department, and, finally, as medical director. During those years, Hunterdon exposed those of us fortunate enough to be a part of her to a panoply of the challenges, problems, and ideas of two decades of change in the health service industry. As I have since traveled around the country, the problems I see in hospital management, mergers, university-community hospital relations, and medical staffs, from OEO health centers to urban centers such as Cook County in Chicago, all are reflected in the Hunterdon experience.

It may be worthwhile to recall the changes which have occurred during these 20 years. In the early 1950s, the interest of foundations and government in upgrading the rural health of this country had faded—all, including academia, were primarily interested in scientific medicine, best expressed by the increasing amounts of support for bench research. The voluntary faculties of the 1940s had disappeared and were replaced by full-time people—thus cutting one viable link between medical town and gown.

As the years passed, we noted an initial recognition that research activity required controls—reflected by mandated explanation to and permission of those subjected to experimentation and by the stricter control of trial pharmaceuticals.

Society slowly recognized the need for improved accessibility and for Federally sponsored fiscal support of our citizens who were not receiving care because of inability to pay. National interest now emphasizes health care application. It was not so in 1950.

Each of us sees Hunterdon from a slightly different perspective. I have always perceived Hunterdon as an experiment in providing total medical and social care, from one source, to the citizens of a precisely defined geographic area. As such, it reflects numerous sub-experiments, each to be tested on its own merits.

Shortly after assuming the role of director, through the generosity of the Commonwealth Fund, three-member teams from the center, consisting of management, board, and medical staff representatives, visited many of those institutions which were also experiments in health organization, such as the Group Health Cooperative of Puget Sound, Kaiser, and Greenwich Hospital in Connecticut. While I'm not sure to what extent we replicated their programs, the visits served to enthuse us all.

At about this time, I visited a friend and professor at one of the affiliated schools. He appeared perplexed that I had accepted the position of medical director and among other things said, "You people have established a nice hospital—now what?" He had struck a rather discordant note, but I need not have been concerned, for the subsequent years brought many challenges. Some—such as the initiation of a home care and a nursing home program, aiding in the formation of a county health board, and developing mental health services—were successful. Others—such as an attempt to develop a milieu for self-evaluation and an attempt to develop a building that housed all health and welfare agencies—were failures.

While it is difficult to discuss one facet of the center's operation without impinging on all others, I would like to describe briefly three of the problem areas and the programs which enfolded in response.

The first is the house staff program, particularly that portion related to the training of family physicians. From its inception, Hunterdon was approved for a one-year general practice residency. We also had arrangements with New York University, the University of Pennsylvania, and Jefferson Medical College for student electives in community medicine. One intern each was rotated from St. Vincent's and Lenox Hill Hospitals in New York City.

With the departure of many of the original directors of service in the late 1950s, it became evident that many of these educational commitments were tenuous at best—often more related to the individuals at each facility than to contractual agreements between institutions. Similarly, the student rotation was unreliable and the number of general practice residents in training each year varied from one to three. This situation was of grave concern since the house staff not only provided needed patient coverage, but stimulated the medical staff and was an integral part of the center's program.

Fortunately, two events occurred which ameliorated the situation. The first was the appointment of two new directors of service in medicine and pediatrics from the University of Pennsylvania. Within a brief time a consistent rotation of students and specialty residents was established with that school and subsequently with others.

Our prime educational commitment, however, had always been the broad training of a new type of family physician, oriented primarily to non-surgical patient care. The second fortuitous event was the report of the Committee on Preparation for General Practice of the American Medical Association in 1959—a report which recognized the need for training a new type of broadly oriented primary care physician. The committee recommended that a minimal and basic two-year pilot program be established to gain experience from which the essentials of a future residency program could be developed.

Through negotiation with the AMA Council on Medical Education and Hospitals we were approved as one of a small number of such pilot educational experiments.

Our program was designed for the two-year period immediately following graduation from medical school—the equivalent of the internship and first year of residency. At Hunterdon the plan involved teaching by the members of all departments and the family physicians. The trainee was exposed to all major areas of medicine including non-operative surgical diagnosis; he followed and cared for patients from the family physician's office to the emergency room to the diagnostic center and the in-patient floors. The social and community aspects of primary care as well as the need for the family physician to interrelate with his specialist peers was emphasized.

In spite of our unique milieu, a glossy brochure, and a very active recruitment program, we attracted no one in the first year. However, in the second and following years the program was more successful, so that during the second half of the 1960s, on several occasions, we had three or four firm applicants for each of the four approved first-year positions.

Together with the other institutions which survived as pilot programs, we participated in the formulation of the essentials and by 1969 were approved for a full three-year family practice residency or 12 residents at a time. Not only did the number of applicants steadily increase, but the quality of the program on more than one occasion attracted men who were at the top of their medical school class—much to the chagrin of some faculty members.

Since the original AMA committee report and the subsequent Millis report, many residencies in family practice have been organized. Some have taken Hunterdon graduates for members of their faculties. A residual problem still exists in many areas—not how to train the primary physician but how to utilize him in a medical system that is specialist-oriented. Hunterdon solved that problem long ago and has demonstrated that the new family physician can perform a central role.

The second event was the development of an incentive program for the full-time specialist staff in 1967.

When the first specialists were employed in 1953–54, each was hired as an individual chief of service at an initial salary of $15,000—without fringe benefits. The definition of their relationship to the center was contained in the center's by-laws and in a brief document describing the professional service fund. The former delineated only their duties as directors of service. From the beginning, meetings of the full-time specialist staff were held, at least monthly, but there was no clear, written definition of how they related to each other or to the center in an organizational sense. From the early years, there was increasing pressure for the development of a quasi-independent group—on two occasions by-laws for the "HMC group" were prepared within the full-time staff meetings, but wiser heads prevailed before the proposals saw the light of day, i.e., were forwarded to the board of trustees. The concept of an organized group was not anathema in itself, but it was inconsistent with the existing center policy. After two years of prolonged discussion, meetings, and writing, a memorandum of agreement was developed (in 1964–65) between each employed physician and the Hunterdon Medical Center, which incorporated all pertinent portions of the by-laws of the medical staff and board, defined the salaries and benefits, and recognized the prevailing practices, such as monthly meetings, etc. At the same time, it developed a set of rules and regulations—familiar to both board and specialists—which could not be amended without the approval of both.

The underlying causes of discontent—leading to the previously described situation—were the low salaries and the policy of equal salary for each specialty director regardless of his income production. These issues arose initially when the first non-director of service was employed and is reflected in the minutes of the specialist staff meetings of that time. The decision was eventually made to treat the new ranks of assistant directors and associates in a similar way to the directors—i.e., all members of each rank receiving equal income but assistant directors $1,000 less basic salary than directors.

As the years passed, differential salaries became a more pressing problem, for while each director had equally defined responsibilities for his department, those on medicine, pediatrics, psychiatry, etc., not only could be expected to produce less income under usual circumstances, but at Hunterdon actually spent a great deal more time supervising family physicians, in-patient care, teaching house staff, etc., far more than the surgical members of the staff.

Each specialist believed he was working to capacity—the surgeons felt that they were supporting those in negative cash flow departments and the non-surgeons believed they were performing non-income producing services, which not only decreased their income but which enabled the surgeons to have house-staff assistance in the operating room. At first, this divisiveness was internecene, but gradually was expressed as dissatisfaction with the "system." As one surgeon who resigned put it, "I see my specialty peers at other places making two to three times my income . . . while I like it here . . . I cannot stay."

The problem of resignations and the inability to acquire replacements became acute and in 1965 the suggestion was made that an incentive program was necessary. Two years later, in 1967, the program was effected. The problem was not the development of a simple incentive related to income production, similar to others around the country, but to maintain a mixture of interest in patient care, teaching, and self-education—basic tenets of the center's program. Productivity and income had to be increased but not at the expense of Hunterdon's comprehensive program.

The incentive plan which was eventually adopted at the

medical center recognized certain principles for the first time:

- That there is a basic difference in the hourly wage of specialties—i.e., surgery and medicine;
- That increased income production merits reward;
- That increased productivity, regardless of income produced, merits reward.

The final plan was basically as follows:

1. Each man's basic salary and fringe benefits are guaranteed.
2. At the end of the year each man's costs (salary, fringe benefits, direct and indirect overhead) are subtracted from his gross billings.
3. If a surplus results, 25% is given directly to the individual as an increase in salary for that year.
4. The remaining 75% of all surpluses remains in the professional service fund to be apportioned to the entire specialist staff by an incentive committee (consisting of three full-time specialists, three trustees, and the medical director) using a point system based on the following six categories.

- Measurable patient care hours (25 points)
- Hours of community activity and continuing education (5 points)
- Administrative responsibilities (15 points)
- Medical center teaching (25 points)
- Attendance at the university (10 points)
- Professional conduct (5 points)

In 1967, the total incentive funds distributed were $100,-046, in 1968 (the first full-incentive year) $204,720.

During the same interval, all five categories of non-income producing hours increased (professional conduct was dropped as a category). For example, in 1967, the total measurable patient-care hours were 11,740, in 1968 they had more than tripled to 39,006.

Clearly, two conclusions can be reached. First, that at least in the Hunterdon milieu equal income regardless of specialty (or work load) was not productive and, second, financial incentive remains a strong motivation for productivity.

The third event I would like to detail was the initiation of a satellite health center in a peripheral area of the county.

For a number of years, we were convinced that the medical center provided in-patient medical care of excellence to the people of Hunterdon County. We were much less sanguine (and this was borne out by patient origin statistics) that we provided ambulant out-patient care to a major portion of the population. The causes of this dichotomy were fairly clear: in peripheral areas, patients followed previously established habit patterns, seeking health care outside the county in which family physicians were few or non-existent. Several county regions where the rate of indigency was highest had the fewest physicians. One such area was the city of Lambertville and its environs, 12 miles from the center, located on the New Jersey shore of the Delaware River. In 1960, Flemington and Clinton, between which the center is located, had one family physician for approximately every 1,000 persons and Lambertville and High Bridge, located at some distance from the hospital, had one family physician for approximately every 2,000 persons. Flemington had 0.9% of its population receiving categorical assistance and Lambertville 2.7%.

Many ineffective attempts were made to convince young family doctors to practice in the least covered areas but to no avail. Not only were they more distant from the stimulation of the medical center but these areas had the reputation of a high indigency rate and poor schools.

We had searched for other answers to the problem of bringing good medical care to all citizens and had come to the belief that peripheral health satellites might be the answer. There were other reasons for our interest in a satellite:

First, an initial satellite would be the beginning of a truly county-wide regional system—at first, a central hospital with peripheral satellites and later, as the county population grew, a large central hospital with smaller peripheral hospitals—all with one board and one staff. The result would be a Hunterdon experiment that was locked in county-wide.

Second, if the satellite was staffed by full-time, salaried family physicians they would become more involved in solving nagging problems of medical management between family doctor and specialist.

There were three regular meetings involving various physicians each month. The full medical staff, the medical board (with equal representation by family physician and specialist), and the full-time specialist staff. The latter contained all the directors and assistant directors of services, and all had common interests, both medical and financial. This is where the power base for medical/administrative decisions lay.

While the relationship between the family physician and specialist was generally quite good, a number of recurrent problems were clear. For example, the original concept in obstetrics (as with other departments) was that the family doctor would be responsible for pre- and post-partum care and for "normal," uncomplicated obstetrical deliveries. The obstetrician would be available for consultation, surgery, and referrals. In fact, the previously established family doctors gave up obstetrics one by one and the newer physicians, as they established successful practices, did the same. The "normal" obstetrical load of the specialists increased each year much to their displeasure. On the other hand, an ever larger proportion of the obstetricians' out-patient practice was taken up by routine six- and twelve-month pelvic examinations, which were arranged outside the usual referral pattern between patient and gynecologist—usually without the family physician's knowledge.

These and similar problems had been discussed ad infinitum at medical board, medical staff, and in special sessions with the professional affairs committee of the board of trustees. Some of us believed that if satellite family MDs were added to the full-time staff and paid from the professional fund, common fiscal and medical interests would devise new solutions—more representative of both groups.

The third reason for our interest in the satellite program was that it would firm up the full-time specialty system. Outside specialists (not interested in Hunterdon as an experiment) would tend to enter the county only if there were areas of vacuum in medical coverage. Also, since we could not be accused of failing to render service to a specific area, suits from excluded physicians, if they occurred, would have less chance of success.

Fourth, the satellite would be an effective adjunct to medical center training programs, particularly for family practice residents and for para-professionals.

We were not sure how to stimulate and finance the first such project until correspondence occurred between the Hunterdon board and the Phillips Memorial Hospital in Lambertville. The latter had been incorporated in 1920 following the wishes expressed in the will of Edgar T. Phillips— to construct and endow a hospital in Lambertville and to support the indigent sick in the area. Unfortunately, the will's funds were insufficient for those purposes, and for several decades the Phillips Fund had contributed to rescue squads, area hospitals, and the indigent sick. With the advent of Medicare and other sources of support for the needy ill, the trustees of the fund had become concerned as to the future use of their monies while at the same time carrying out the wishes of Mr. Phillips and Mr. Barber, from whom the fund had received additional monies in 1939.

In 1966, after consideration of other possibilities, the Phillips board asked the medical center to study their problem and make appropriate recommendations. The study was completed and recommendations made in a report to the

Phillips board. The essentials of that report have since been implemented. The Phillips board presented eight acres of land to the medical center and provided the necessary funds to erect a modern and very attractive community health center which was placed in operation with two full-time family physicians and was named the Phillips-Barber Family Health Center of the Hunterdon Medical Center. The building contains space for basic laboratory and X ray services, for small public meetings, for health nursing, etc.

This satellite placed the health services of Lambertville in a regional complex of medical care which included the central medical center and its affiliated universities. Hopefully, it has filled the previously noted vacuum of ambulatory care in that peripheral area of the county.

I hope that these three episodes in the life of the Hunterdon Medical Center have indicated the viability and continued imagination of the organization.

Opinion on how medical care should be provided in the United States has become an emotional and political issue. Many seem to cling to specific ideas as general panaceas to all health and social problems. The Kaiser experience, for example, has had great appeal—particularly its pre-paid insurance component which has been blessed for cutting costs and decreasing inappropriate utilization of costly in-patient facilities. For many years Hunterdon's utilization statistics for Blue Cross and Blue Shield patients compared favorably with those published by Kaiser. However, we were not working under a pre-paid umbrella—the two organizations' obvious similarities were adequate available ambulatory facilities and a framework of peer discipline and supervision. I believe the latter is the important operational constraint to inappropriate utilization.

In recent years, we have heard of increasing Kaiser Plan costs and utilization, and at the same time evidence is accumulating that similar utilization experience is noted when better controls, particularly by regional peers, are imposed on hospital care. The pre-payment concept may not be a panacea after all.

Neither is Hunterdon a panacea. However, three needs appear self-evident nationally. *Delivery of care must be well organized*—the Hunterdon program is as organized on a truly geographic level as any other plan. *Health services must be available to all*—Hunterdon has made this a basic premise since its inception and has strived to fulfill its responsibility. *There must be better control, by peers, of inappropriate or unnecessary care*—Hunterdon's response is reflected in its utilization statistics.

I believe that the changes that we will note in health care delivery during the next two decades will be equally exciting as those of the past 20 years. For example, there is much activity, particularly in the academic milieu, in training "new" types of health workers to cut costs, to improve availability, and to relieve the physician of his "overburden." While these motives may be appropriately altruistic, they are dissimilar to pressures that have changed medical manpower in the past.

In 1900, physicians made up 63% of the direct providers of health care. They constituted 23% of the group in 1970. Technological and scientific advances played a significant role in these shifts of work loads and manpower requirements, and the rate of technological discovery in health care appears to be increasing. Decreasing costs of computers in medicine and of two-way high resolution television, improvements in telemetry and the further development of the picture phone —all these will have a marked effect both on the nature of health care delivery and the character of new paramedical types.

These and other developments should challenge the Hunterdon Medical Center, occupied in maximizing medical care to its citizens over the next two decades. I believe that the center will meet the challenge.

HUNTERDON TODAY

•

Frederick J. Knocke, M.D.
(Medical Director, 1971–   )

Hunterdon Medical Center continues to adhere to its basic goal, namely, to provide the best possible medical service in Hunterdon County, to be the center of health care for the community. Previous speakers have outlined our philosophy, how it was developed, and how we have attempted to implement it, our successes, and our failures. We continue to provide for the delivery of family-oriented care in the patient's neighborhood by competent (Board certified or Board eligible in family practice) doctors, backed by appropriate specialists and technical facilities, a modern hospital, and support services with potential for outreach into the community.

The medical center, which had 106 beds when it opened, now has 195 beds with a spectrum of care from coronary and intensive care to in-patient ambulatory services.

Our staff consists of 25 family doctors with offices in the community and 34 full-time specialists, based in the hospital.

The specialties represented are internal medicine (sub-specialties—cardiology, gastroenterology, hematology, rheumatology and metabolic diseases, and chest diseases), pediatrics, general surgery (with a sub-specialty in vascular surgery), obstetrics and gynecology, orthopaedics, urology, ophthalmology, otolaryngology, oral surgery, psychiatry, dermatology, anesthesiology, pathology, and radiology.

In-patient care is often followed up by an active home

care program which is hospital directed. Ancillary services include social service, physical medicine—including physical therapy and occupational therapy, speech and hearing, and dietary counselling—and standard hospital operating departments.

A recent New Jersey Department of Health listing faulted us for not having clinics which coincide with the in-patient services we now provide. Hunterdon is proud of its concept that all patients are cared for on the basis of medical need, regardless of ability to pay, both in the doctor's office and in the hospital. This eliminates the necessity of separating patients into clinic patients on the basis of economic background and ensures a single, high standard of medical care.

To help bring primary care to some underserved parts of the county, the hospital has acquired land in three separate areas. On two of these, doctors' offices and support areas have been constructed and staffed—our satellite program.

In Lambertville, the staffing is by two full-time family physicians who are on the hospital payroll, and in Clinton the building is rented to two independent family practitioners. In each case, hospital facilities such as social service, physical therapy, lab, and X ray will be phased into these satellites as the need arises. Eventually, as the county grows, in-patient beds can also be included. We plan to do this before the present hospital becomes so large that it becomes fragmented and difficult to manage as a unit.

An active teaching program is essential to keep the staff intellectually stimulated and to ensure trained personnel who will stay and work in the community. The residency program in family practice, among the seven first approved by the AMA Council on Medical Education as described by Dr. Henderson, has expanded to 18 positions, six appointed each year to our three-year program. The fact that it is a quality program is attested by the fact that we had 84 applications for the six positions in the matching program last year, and inquiries this year are running ahead of last year. Eighteen of the 25 family physicians practicing in Hunterdon at present went through our residency training program.

Graduate medical education for family doctors is centered in the fact that all patients admitted to the hospital are part of the teaching program, being worked up by the house staff and reviewed on rounds with the full-time staff. There is, therefore, an interplay of information between the attending family doctor, the house staff, and the full-time specialist staff. Family doctors may admit patients under their own care to the medical and pediatric services, for normal obstetrics, and for minor surgical procedures. By bringing the family doctor into the hospital, his patients receive continuity of care, and he benefits from the stimulation of working with the house staff and attending staff in the hospital environment. Teaching centered around the doctor's own patient is an excellent way to provide continuing education.

This spectrum of teaching (undergraduate, house staff, and graduate education for the attending staff) takes time— 8,000 to 10,000 hours each year—contributed by the specialist staff. Who pays for this teaching? A portion is contributed by the teacher in return for his academic appointment, for having the house staff to help care for his patients, and because he likes to teach. A portion should be paid by the patient and by his third party insurance carrier, because he gets better patient care in a hospital with a good teaching program. And a portion should be supported by the community and state because a teaching program insures a continuing supply of well-qualified practitioners for the community.

In nursing, we cooperate with Somerset Community College to provide clinical experience for their students who earn an associate degree in nursing. The local Hunterdon Central Regional High School in Flemington offers a two-year practical nurse training program, involving the senior year of high school and one additional year of clinical experience which is provided at Hunterdon Medical Center. Several schools of nursing observe our maternity operation which, for many years, has encouraged the husbands to be in the delivery room with their wives during delivery. A nursing aid training course for selected inmates of the New Jersey State Prison for Women at Clinton is based at the hospital and has been quite successful as part of their vocational rehabilitation program. The radiology department runs a state-approved course in radiologic technology, with eight students, four enrolled each year. In pathology, a one-year course for clinical laboratory assistants trains four technicians annually.

Affiliation with a medical school ensures continuing contact with academic medicine, and is essential to prevent professional stagnation. This was one of the cornerstones of our original organization. For many years our contract was with New York University. Two years ago, as New York University became more concerned with central city problems, we negotiated a new affiliation with the New Jersey College of Medicine and Dentistry-Rutgers Medical School, and this was signed early in 1972. Because of close ties between the medical school and the hospital, the director of the Hunterdon Medical Center is a member, with vote, of the executive faculty committee of the medical school, and his appointment is a joint one by the board of trustees of Hunterdon Medical Center and the New Jersey College of Medicine and Dentistry-Rutgers Medical School.

All of our full-time specialist staff have academic clinical appointments at the school and are actively involved in teaching programs. With the expansion of the department of family practice at the medical school, it is anticipated that many of our family practitioners will also be appointed to the clinical staff of the medical school.

The hospital is actively involved in the Rutgers undergraduate training program, and is responsible for a third of the primary clinical training of the third-year medical school class particularly in the departments of medicine, surgery, obstetrics and gynecology, psychiatry, and pediatrics. Physical diagnosis instruction and experience in the department of pathology is provided for second-year students. We also offer several fourth-year clerkships which are open to students from Rutgers and other medical schools.

It is now almost four years since I assumed responsibility for the direction of Hunterdon Medical Center. My time is devoted about 75 percent to administration, but I continue to practice my specialty of orthopaedic surgery for the remainder of the time.

Management of the institution is implemented with the support of a team of assistant directors, one each for medical affairs, hospital administration, financial management, nursing, and data processing. Hunterdon has always been directed by a physician because of its unusual medical staffing patterns, and because the basic concern of the board of trustees has been the delivery of medical care to the community as a whole, rather than the mechanics of running a hospital.

During the past four years, the hospital has continued to expand in response to the medical needs of the community. Early in 1971, it was becoming apparent that there was need to expand our medical-surgical bed capacity, and also that our mechanical support systems were inadequate for the ever-enlarging physical plant. At the February 1971 meeting of the board of trustees, we voted to build a one-story, 40-bed, in-patient facility for ambulatory patients over the out-patient parking lot, with the foundation designed to support four additional floors which will be added when more space is required in the ambulatory care wing. A separate power plant was also planned during this expansion. Financial support for these additions was achieved through one of the last Hill-Burton hospital construction grants, by generous support from the George K. Large Foundation, by continuing community support, and by sizeable borrowing.

This expansion was accomplished with a contract manager rather than the usual general contractor. The result was that the final cost was appreciably under estimate, the power plant was operational in October 1972, and the new extended care wing was fully equipped and ready to open in January 1973. This increased our bed capacity to 195 beds from 155 beds.

The Phillips-Barber Family Health Center of the Hunterdon Medical Center opened in 1970 in Lambertville, in the southern part of the county. At first, it was in a renovated doctor's office in town and in September 1972, in a modern office building on the edge of town, donated by a local philanthropic foundation.

In May of 1973, a second office was opened at the North Hunterdon satellite in Clinton, where two doctors rent space and conduct their practices. This will give us the opportunity to compare the delivery of services and the teaching load in a privately run office against one that is hospital-affiliated.

A third area of the county that is underserved medically is the southwest corner centering in Milford and Frenchtown. Thirty acres of land were purchased in Milford in 1972, for construction of a third satellite. Because of fiscal restraints, recruiting problems, and pending definition of need, the hospital has accepted the offer of the use of a building on the site of the Riegel Paper Company in Milford. It is planned to equip, staff, and open this unit in July 1974.

This satellite program serves a dual purpose: First, to bring medical care with the support of ancillary hospital facilities to areas of the county which would otherwise be underserved; second, it provides the model family practice units necessary for the residency training program.

Our mental health program has expanded through the years. With the help of Federal, state, and private financial support, a 14-bed in-patient service, day care and night care center, and an extensive out-patient mental health center opened in January 1972. The program has been supported with a Federal staffing grant, and the staff has been expanded to include three psychiatrists, three psychologists, four psychiatric social workers, one full-time pastoral counsellor, and one full-time clinical nursing specialist. Programs include a methadone program and alcoholism information center.

Our home health service has been expanded with the addition of a full-time nurse director, and our new director of nursing, Eleanor Claus, who assumed her duties in June 1973, has a strong background in community nursing in addition to training in nursing administration. This service encourages early discharge from the hospital, with continuing care in the patient's home. It contracts with the Family Nursing Service of Hunterdon County for home nursing care and with the Homemakers Service for housekeeping help until the patient can manage these responsibilities himself. Hospital ancillary services, such as physical medicine, social service, and speech and hearing are also available to the patient at home.

Mr. Wescott outlined our early interest in establishing a pre-paid payment plan for medical care in Hunterdon County which was abandoned because it did not seem possible in 1953. However, the interest remained, and in 1969 and 1970 the time seemed right to reassess the possibility of working out a plan for pre-paid medical care for Hunterdon County. Dr. Henderson and Mr. Wescott approached the Commonwealth Fund and a $31,000 grant for a feasibility study was obtained in 1970. The initial investigation was undertaken with the help of the Leonard Davis Institute of Health Economics of the University of Pennsylvania and the Prudential Insurance Company. The results were favorable and in the spring of 1971, when the Federal government (Department of Health, Education, and Welfare) became more actively interested in this phase of the delivery of medical care and set up funds for HMO (Health Maintenance Organization) grants, the basic work had been done. Dr. Avrum Labe Katcher compiled a grant request which was approved on June 19, 1971, and funded for $99,600. This was a planning grant. The Leonard Davis Institute continued in a consultative role. The Prudential Insurance Company made available to us several very knowledgeable members of its staff.

Detailed, elaborate plans for administration, financing, data processing, and marketing were formulated.

In the early stages, it appeared that cooperation of the professional staff, both specialists and family doctors, would be obtained, but as the planning progressed and a final plan was proposed, more and more questions were raised by the physicians. These questions centered about payment mechanisms, fiscal risk assumed by the doctors, and how much the delivery of medical care would be stifled by government regulation and red tape.

Concern about these and related questions became so marked that at a meeting on March 22, 1972, the staff voted 2 to 1 against participating in the plan as proposed.

Despite some efforts by the combined citizen and doctor Hunterdon Health Plan Board of Trustees no further progress has been made towards implementing a health maintenance organization. Hopefully, some means of implementing a pre-paid plan for the citizens of Hunterdon will be worked out in the future, a plan that would respond to the providers' reservations, and still enable the citizens of our community to benefit financially from the efficiencies of the Hunterdon system of delivery of medical care.

How to financially reward our full-time staff is a continuing challenge. In recent years, there has been increasing unrest and dissatisfaction with the various incentive formulas, which were repeatedly revised to recognize the various contributions of the different departments and members of the full-time staff. From the first, the agreement between the doctors and the hospital was that the doctors would charge fees for service and that the money earned would go into a separate fund (the professional service fund) which would not be subsidized by the hospital, and which, in turn, would not support hospital operations. In practice, this is rather complicated to administer, since the hospital provides the physical plant, in the past in exchange for teaching, administration, etc. Management and business office functions, record keeping, personnel services, these are provided by the hospital and must be paid for. Since these are integrated into the total hospital operation and accounting system, they frequently are at variance with the wishes of the individual physician and his ideas of what would be the most efficient operation of his department. Compromises must be reached —for example, a unit record system maintained and mandated by the hospital for all in- and out-patients versus separate records available in the doctor's office for active out-patients.

Finally, how is it possible to weigh the contribution of one member with a high patient care load versus one with high teaching and administrative responsibilities? How to recognize income generation, and the marketplace for the various specialties? The incentive committee has been unable to come up with a plan that equitably recognizes these various factors and few of the members were satisfied with the result.

To respond to these pressures, recompense in 1974 will be on the basis of a pre-negotiated sum for each department. This figure will be arrived at by mutually determining appropriate work load, teaching responsibilities, expected revenue, and considering the national income figures in the various specialties. Hopefully, it will work better than the original plan of equal salary for equal position, or the constantly shifting incentive plans of the past few years.

Finally, what are some of the issues of particular concern at the moment? Our 20-year-old plant is now serving twice the population for which it was originally designed. Immediate needs are a new emergency room, new operating rooms, and an expanded radiology department.

Population will undoubtedly expand at an ever-increasing rate and the nature of the county will change from rural to suburban. In long range plans, changing patterns of care must be considered, i.e., out-patient surgery, shorter lengths of stay, change in patient mix as our understanding and treatment methods of major diseases improve. A medical breakthrough in cancer control might have the same effect on OR and surgical beds as the pill had on delivery rooms and occupancy on the obstetrical floor.

Quality control, documentation of patterns of care, utilization by diagnosis, analysis of cost per disease category, all are increasingly mandated. PSROs (Professional Standards Review Organizations) are around the corner. We must plan along these lines.

How does a hospital stay fiscally viable in these days of increasing government restraint and control? We are squeezed between one division of the New Jersey Department of Health which tells us to expand services, and another which tells us to cut costs in the same area. A Federal government with mandated guidelines places a strait jacket on our fiscal operation. More and more ingenuity is required to come up with innovations to improve care and cut costs in the increasingly restrictive arena in which medical care is being delivered.

Because of the constraints, in this year of the 200th anniversary of the Boston Tea Party, I more and more sympathize with the hardy and independent colonists, who responded to increasing government restraints and taxation by dumping the symbol of that oppression into Boston harbor.

If we were to dump all the government regulations, red tape, and computer printouts relative to health care into Boston harbor, the poor city of Boston would be isolated from the sea, its harbor choked with a sodden mass of paper waste.

Barring revolution, we shall have to work within the system. For the future, we remain committed to the delivery of care to the entire community as economically and efficiently as we can. The basis of our system remains the family practitioner in the community supported by the hospital-based specialist. Our teaching efforts are important, and are focused on training in the specialty of family practice. Ancillary medical services are stressed, both in hospital and in outreach programs. We shall try to continue to respond in innovative and effective ways to the ever-changing needs for medical services in Hunterdon County.

PART II

Hunterdon Medical Center
Underlying Concepts

THE FAMILY PHYSICIAN AND THE HUNTERDON MEDICAL CENTER

●

Hiram B. Curry, M.D.

For many years I have heard good things about the Hunterdon Medical Center. When I was a solo general practitioner in Jasper, Florida, I read about this forward-thinking group and your experiment to provide superior health care to all the people of Hunterdon County. I must confess that my perception of health care at that time was very narrow and perhaps myopic. The Hunterdon plan seemed too futuristic to work. My interest was no more than casual until 1968, when I became concerned that our medical profession was doing a very poor job of translating current knowledge and skills into medical and health service. After meeting Dr. Frank Snope and Dr. William Willard in 1970 and hearing more about Hunterdon, my interest in this medical center became keen. Soon I recognized that Hunterdon is one of our finest models for providing comprehensive health care.

This occasion has afforded me the opportunity to read about the planning and the establishment of the Hunterdon Medical Center. As I read, I became involved and was compelled to arrive one day early to tour the facility and to talk with the doctors in order to understand the full scope of your enterprise. I can report today that my expectations have been exceeded in every way. Indeed, you have a center which has been well planned. I congratulate the early planners on their resolve to have a health center that would solve more problems than an ordinary county hospital. Their vision included comprehensive care with continuity, care delivered with human concern, for all the citizens of Hunterdon County.

Those same words express the wishes of the leaders of general practice in the 1950s as they pondered their diminishing number and the increasing work load placed on the remaining ones. The makeshift episodic care of the past clearly would not be a satisfactory pattern for the future. Comprehensive care delivered with continuity and in a personal manner became the by-words of the late 1960s for the new specialty of family practice, then in a fetal stage. Clearly, there was a yearning, even a determination, to develop a specialty that could better serve the patient, his family, and his community, and merit the respect of other specialists.

The remarks made so far today and the entire setting of this meeting make me wish to review for you the difference between general practice and family practice. In the past the general practitioner, armed only with the knowledge and skills he learned in medical school and during his internship, opened his office and rendered service to the public. General practitioners in the past have not had the opportunity for careful preparation for their work. They have had to learn on their own to be effective practitioners through on-the-job experience. Most general practices provide episodic remedial care after a person has an illness or a problem. In the general practice of the past there has been a lack of planning for health care.

Some general practitioners have grown remarkably with their experience, for every year in the field there has been a year's growth. A general practitioner with 25 years' experience is a very valuable man in his community. I regret to say that not all general practitioners have grown so.

The forward-thinking doctors who were concerned in the 1950s with the ever diminishing number of general practitioners sought specialty status for general practice as a means to upgrade this medical vocation and to attract more students into this field. Because general practice did not represent a unique body of knowledge and did not claim responsibility for rendering a unique service to society, it was denied specialty status. After carefully analyzing the services rendered by the very best of the general practitioners, concerned medical leaders realized that the tenured family doctor's knowledge of family psychodynamics allows him to understand complaints at a greater depth than most specialists and enables him to work effectively caring for the entire family. In February 1969, the American Medical Association Council on Medical Education acknowledged that health care for all members of the family, regardless of age, did represent a special responsibility and required a unique body of knowledge. Therefore, the council granted board specialty status.

The wedge is one of our oldest tools. Allow me to use it as a model to explain one of our oldest professions. (Figure 1) In the past, we have learned in our medical schools a great deal about cells, organs, and tissues, and diseases which affect these structures. On the whole, medical schools have done a fine job teaching us the anatomy and the physiology of our bodies, the diseases which may affect us, and pharmacology which may be applied to correct the faults. A great deal of attention has been directed to our physical bodies and their frailties.

Our society has organized certain health services and health-related programs to insure attention to many general problems and care for some identified groups. We have these health services organized at national, state, county, and even city levels. The educational efforts of our medical schools and the efforts of society do not join comfortably to furnish us an efficient system that meets the needs of our society. Something is missing.

Psychiatry has blossomed in the past 30 years, focusing attention on the diseases which can affect our minds. Special attention has been given to the major psychoses and the major mental illnesses. Much less attention has been focused on the neuroses and behavioral abnormalities which mar the health of so many. Only recently have a few ministers and ethicists joined the faculties of a few medical schools to encourage

FIGURE 1

Cell
Organ
System
Disease
City
County
District
State
Nation

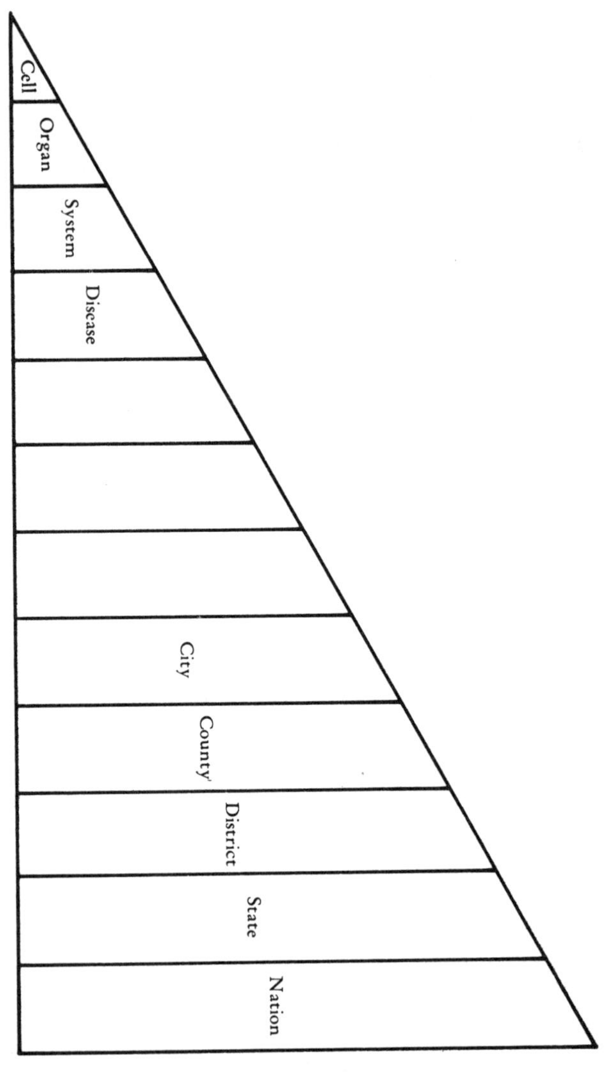

discussion of guilt feelings and debate of ethical issues in medicine. At last we have combined the physical, the mental, and even the spiritual aspects of man—the whole person. At first glance, this seems to represent great progress. Before we congratulate ourselves, let us pause and realize that we have just described a hermit. (Figure 2) The medical care provided by Hunterdon Medical Center and its Phillips-Barber Family Health Center in Lambertville has not been designed for the care of hermits. What more, then, is needed for the care of these patients? What is the difference between a hermit and a human? What is the difference between a male individual and a man, husband, or a father? I believe it is one of relationships. The relationships that each of us has with parents, spouse, children, and friends makes each of us human. It is the early orientation that sets the course for one's life. It is the intrafamily relationship, or bonds of love, between the members of the family that is to influence future relationships with others, one's sense of personal identity, and ultimately one's sense of well-being and fulfillment. The unique concern of family practice is the understanding of the patient in his family setting, the understanding of the dynamics of the family, and how both of these contribute to the over-all health and happiness of the person. (Figure 3)

Where there is a relationship, there is a behavioral interaction. Now we are considering the behavior of the person. It is behavior which makes him human. Behavior makes each of us different and unique. In the past, medical science has stressed the physical and mental aspects of man. Only recently has it begun to focus attention on behavior and the effects of behavior on our health. The total of all the viral and bacterial invasions of the body which result in infections, all the degenerative changes of blood vessels and joints which affect the body, the wild growth of cells which result in cancer, and all the other "organic" maladies that affect our bodies, the total is less than half of human complaints. The tensions, the anxieties, the fears, the disquietude of mind, and the dis-eases

FIGURE 2

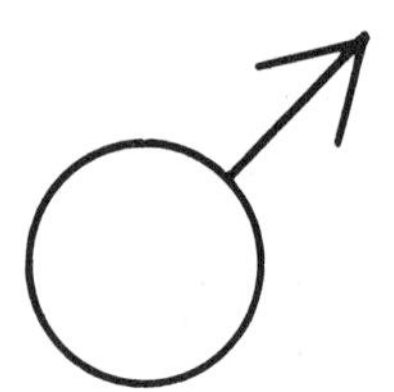

FIGURE 3

A FAMILY

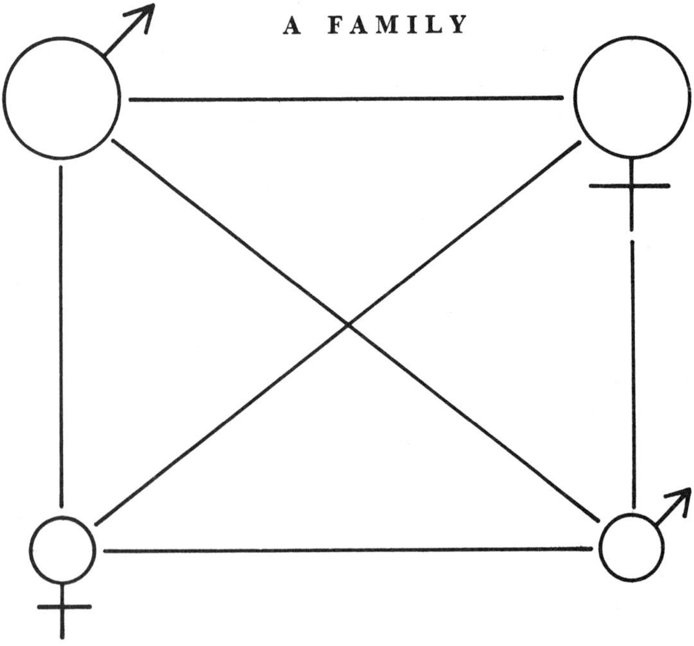

of body that result from faulty or abnormal relationships, all modify our behavior and cause us to enjoy life less than we should.

The best of the general practitioners of the past who have served the members of families over a period of years gained intuitively an understanding of these relationships and used this knowledge effectively to accurately appraise the medical and health problems of the family. This understanding developed as he served the family members and observed their behavior over a period of years.

The tenured position of the family doctor results in a doctor-patient relationship in which the patient trusts the doctor and the doctor is devoted to his patient. As this trusting relationship develops, the patient's guard is let down. Not only is a more adequate and more accurate history given, but the accompanying feelings which are very important are also revealed. The family doctor is able to use this relationship as a reliable diagnostic tool because it helps uncover information and as a powerful therapeutic agent because of the trust it engenders. It is important for our modern family physicians to understand both the relationship between and among family members and his own relationship with each member of the family and the family as a whole.

A tremendous amount of information about human behavior has been collected, analyzed, and structured as a science —behavioral science—by psychologists and behavioral and social scientists. These scientists are able to teach us much more about human behavior in a short period than would result from years of personal observation, even if we grew with every experience. Behavioral science is stressed in our family practice programs. The subject is too important to leave to chance and observation. It is our aim for young family physicians to use their position, the relationship they enjoy with their patients, their personalities, as well as their medical knowledge in the care of their patients.

I am very pleased to see you give careful attention to behavioral science in the training of family physicians here at Hunterdon. You are using modern tools, both the television camera and video-taping equipment, to provide reliable feedback to residents, affording them the opportunity to profit from their errors and to be properly rewarded for their triumphs. I predict behavioral science will receive even greater attention in your training program in the future.

Before we leave the whole person and the family, I wish to say that I believe the family is the biological and social unit of man's living. I also believe one cannot understand the individual as a human unless one looks at him in the context of the family. Neither can one understand the family as a unit of living unless one looks at it in the context of the community. Perhaps a nomad family in the Sahara Desert lives as an isolated family. In our society, groups of families live together and develop relationships with each other and with relatives and friends. Families also develop relationships with churches and schools, with industry, and with other organizations which serve the needs of families within the community. This larger unit of living requires a wider view of health. (Figure 4) The man whose income is inadequate to meet the needs of his family must have feelings of inadequacy and guilt that prevent him from enjoying and experiencing life fully. This can be the cause of many complaints and diseases. Now we can see how the community can affect the health of its constituent families and the individuals in them. The new science of community medicine is young. Here in Hunterdon County where your center serves a defined population, you may have a unique opportunity to help develop this new science and to show all of us how community medicine can improve health care for families and individuals.

I was very favorably impressed by the health records in your Lambertville satellite. There the records are filed by families. The files contain a careful indexing of the medical complaints and health problems of the entire community. You are well on your way toward establishing a data base which will

FIGURE 4

A COMMUNITY

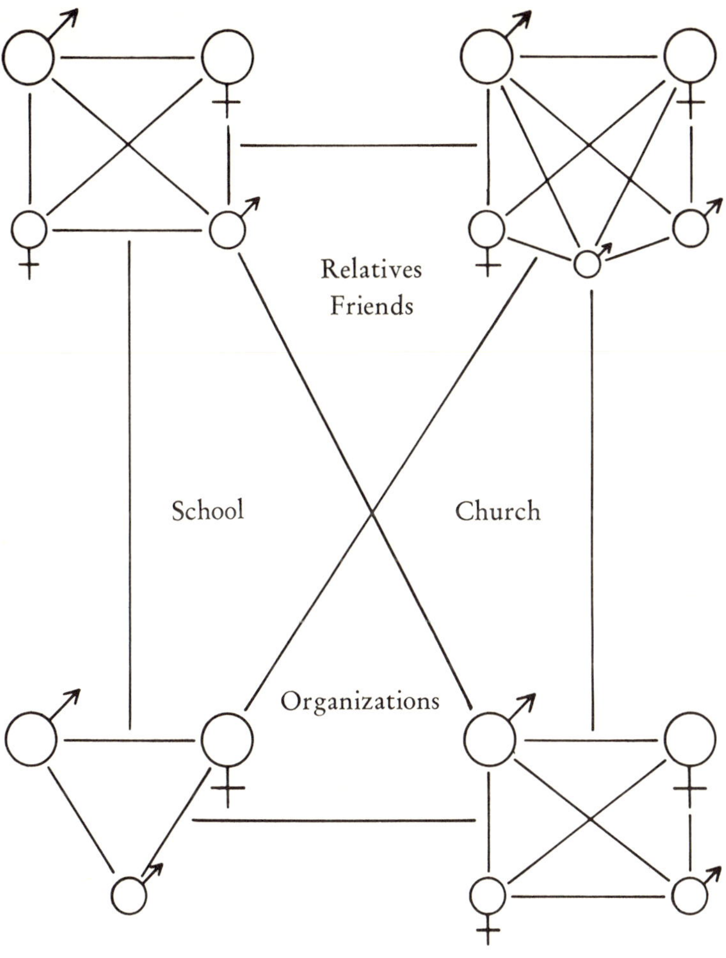

include both disease entities and health hazards in your community. Not only is this information extremely valuable for health care but this data is also very useful for research purposes. Most of the health data for our nation have been derived from severely ill patients in the hospitals, predominantly in large hospitals. The data base currently available is not representative of the medical and health problems of the American people. Clearly, we need a valid data base, one which includes the care given in doctors' offices, clinics, and small hospitals if we are to be able to plan wisely for our country's future health care. The record system you have and the data you are collecting here in Hunterdon County provide a good model for us. I urge you to be even more diligent in your collection of health data for its importance extends far beyond your county borders.

By focusing attention on the whole man, appreciating that he must be understood as a human; on the family, seeing it as the social and biological unit of living; and on the community, the unit of societal living; and by training doctors who can implement these concepts, we can meet the health manpower needs of our nation. These doctors, trained as I have outlined, will be able to relate to the health resources provided by society better than those trained in the traditional pattern. Our wedge is complete. Every interface in our model can be a site for activity and development and a source of strength. I believe our profession can be as strong and useful as the wedge. I believe family practice offers in its concepts and service a means by which medical education and the medical profession can more adequately meet the needs and expectations of society. (Figure 5)

I like the way you have organized the physicians in your center and its satellites. From the very beginning, you have accorded your family physicians an essential position in your county and in your hospital. In some health centers, the family physician has been excluded from the hospital, assigned to work only in his office. My observations strongly suggest

FIGURE 5

Cell
Organ
System
Disease
Whole Person
Family
Com-munity
City
County
District
State
Nation

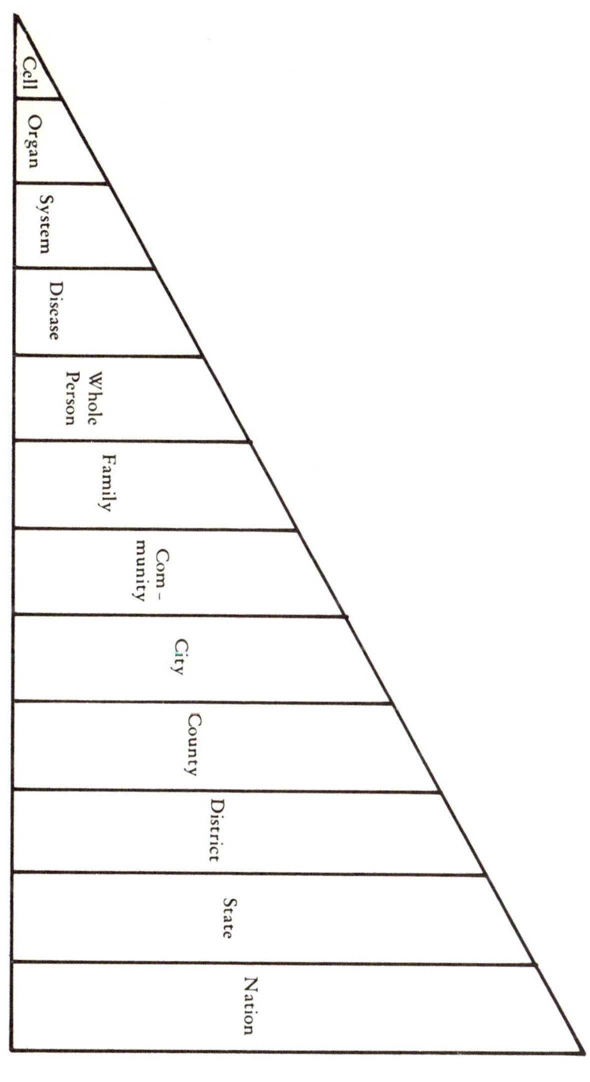

to me that the family physician needs the stimulation of working with challenging problems which require hospitalization and to exchange ideas with other physicians in the hospital. In some areas, specialists in hospitals have looked down their noses at family doctors and failed to recognize their competence to manage many problems in the hospital. When this has occurred, the opportunity for mutual support and growth and the opportunity for superior health care for the people and the community has been missed.

The early planners of the Hunterdon Medical Center included the family physicians, all the family physicians in the county, from the very beginning. They realized that many hospitalized patients would require competent consultants. In order to accord the consultants their proper role, they were made responsible for quality care of the disease process for which the patient was admitted to the hospital. The same policy is operative today. The family physician remains in charge of the patient as long as he is competent to do so, and the staff consultant makes rounds and utilizes the patient for teaching. In this manner the patient receives the very finest care available. The information known by the family physician is available for the care of the patient, and the expertise of the consultant is available to help solve the medical problem. In addition, the patient's illness is utilized for the instruction of family practice residents and for the continuing education of practicing family physicians. When the illness of the patient is complex, the consultant assumes the responsibility and the family physician follows in tandem. I understand this arrangement continues today throughout the hospital except in obstetrics where the limited number of family physicians and the wishes of society have required the obstetrician to function as a primary physician.

The wisdom of the early planners of the Hunterdon Medical Center again shows through in their linking the center with medical schools. The rotation of residents through the center provides stimulus for continued growth of the staff and creates an additional learning opportunity at another level. Medical students from medical schools stimulate and enrich the learning climate for any institution.

It seems that Hunterdon County has separated primary, secondary, and tertiary medical care more clearly than any other delivery system I know. This affords me the opportunity to comment on primary medical care. Many people glibly talk about family practice physicians, internists, and pediatricians as being primary physicians. These persons apparently have forgotten that primary physicians are simply physicians of first contact. General practitioners, family physicians, pediatricians, and internists serve this purpose most often, but the affluent executive may go to a neurosurgeon with his back pain, the affluent housewife to the dermatologist with her rash, the elderly dowager to a professor of hematology when she believes that she is frail and weak. In these instances the highly specialized physician is the primary physician or the physician of first contact. All of us recognize that this is a very inefficient use of our health manpower; but in the American system we have permitted the patient to choose his physician even though the patient may not benefit and the consultant's time may be wasted. So long as we permit the people to choose their physicians, we must be very careful not to misuse the word primary.

The study of relationships within the family and human behavior, and the fact that many human complaints have their origins in faulty relationships and improper behavioral responses constitutes the unique core of family medicine. Just as psychiatry is strongly related to very abnormal behavior, e.g., psychoses, family medicine assumes the responsibility for relationships and behavior which can be dealt with at a more superficial level of understanding. In the past, many problems have been ignored; they have not been severe enough to warrant psychiatric attention, yet they have caused much human misery. The understanding of this body of knowledge and developing requisite skills to deal with these problems is a unique feature of family medicine.

Just as the anesthesiologist is required to know some anatomy, physiology, pathology, and pharmacology pertaining to the heart, so every specialist should be acquainted with the precepts of family medicine. In this way, I believe we can enrich and improve the whole medical profession. It is the responsibility of the family physician to be the master of this subject, and he will utilize it more than other doctors, just as the cardiologist uses information concerning the heart more than other physicians. Inasmuch as Hunterdon County has about 25 family physicians, 18 of whom have been trained in this center and 12 already Board certified, there is an excellent opportunity here to instill these precepts of family medicine into the total practice of medicine. It would be very interesting to query the hospital staff to determine changes in their attitudes which may have resulted from exposure to these family physicians practicing in this community and in this hospital. My prediction is that they have learned much from these family doctors which has resulted in better patient care and more enjoyment in the practice of their specialties.

In the early history of the Hunterdon Medical Center, a very careful study was made of chronic disease in the community. This constitutes a very important health base-line that can now be used to determine the real improvement in your community's health. I realize a repeat study will be very difficult and costly, but the possibility exists here for measuring the increased longevity, the increased ability to work and to enjoy life which has resulted from the establishment of this unique medical center in your community. This community has what many communities are working toward. To do such a study and to prove that this type of organization does indeed contribute to health as measured by these parameters will offer much encouragement to other communities. Here is the opportunity to prove that comprehensive care delivered with continuity and with personal concern is superior to the episodic care of the past. This is a very important challenge. I hope you will seize the opportunity.

One of the great problems facing America today is a data

base for health planning. How many doctors do we need to care for the population? How many family doctors, how many pediatricians and internists are needed for a stated population? What mix of doctors constitutes the most efficient grouping is yet to be decided in this country. Certainly the information available here based on your experience is very valuable. Your mix here in Hunterdon County may well represent the model for the nation for a semi-rural area.

In closing, I wish to congratulate the citizens who had the courage to look at their problem and plan so carefully to solve the health needs of Hunterdon County in such an innovative and creative manner. You have actually increased the number of family doctors in your county while during the same period most counties in the United States have experienced a progressive decline in the number of family physicians. Your family physicians have a real interest in your county as evidenced by the fact that they have returned to the county in which they trained to raise their families and to practice medicine. The quality of your family practice residency program is not disputed. Medical students compete vigorously to have the opportunity to train here. The physicians who have stood the Board examination have performed well, and 12 of your current family physicians are already certified by the American Board of Family Practice. Twenty years ago you had no specialists in this county. Now there are 34 specialists serving this magnificent hospital. Your board of trustees is concerned about the whole population of your county. It has good plans for outreach programs to meet all the people's needs within the county. Your Lambertville program already provides a model for patient care and for health education.

I wish to thank you for inviting me to participate in this symposium. It has been an educational experience for me. I am confident many of the things I have seen and learned here will be translated into changes in our program in South Carolina.

A FULL-TIME HOSPITAL MEDICAL STAFF: PROBLEMS AND PROSPECTS

●

Samuel Wolfe, M.D.

Hunterdon County and Flemington, New Jersey, are well known to informed persons around the world who are concerned about unmet needs for health care and services, and about how one community developed an approach to rationalize the organization of medical practice for an entire county, and at the same time attempted to redefine the roles and relationships of specialists to one another and to the family doctors in the community.

It is especially gratifying to me to see here today two of my not-so-very-old mentors, Dr. Ray E. Trussell, who when he was Dean of Columbia's School of Public Health helped to teach me to think more rationally about health care issues and arranged for my first visit to Hunterdon, and Dr. Jack Elinson, who taught me the little I know about health care research and evaluation, and whose pioneer work (along with Dr. Trussell) in Hunterdon County, *Chronic Illness in a Rural Area: The Hunterdon Study** about the county's unmet needs for care and services, remains the key benchmark study in its field.

It is worthwhile to repeat the four concepts that determined the Hunterdon program:

    1. That the family doctor is an essential element of the health care team;

* Cambridge, Mass.: Harvard University Press, 1959.

2. That the specialties would be provided by a closed, full-time, salaried staff practicing under the hospital—the Hunterdon Medical Center roof—and, in principle, accepting the county's patients only from the family doctors;

3. That the hospital would take initiatives to provide a broad spectrum of health services to the entire county; and

4. That the hospital would have a medical school affiliation and be directly involved in teaching.

I am going to try to deal, briefly, with three questions given below:

1. Do or do not the core problems that are divisive within a full-time hospital-based staff of medical specialists relate primarily to the question of money?

2. What are the prospects for the continued stability of the Hunterdon Medical Center concept of salaried, full-time specialists in the next two decades?

3. If the Hunterdon County experiment has been so great, why has it not moved from being an atypical experiment to being emulated in scores of other settings in the United States?

I start with several assumptions that are, I think, rather well proved about what makes the Hunterdon health services good. First, hospitals with very highly structured medical staff organizations, such as Hunterdon, are of better quality than are hospitals that are very loosely structured. Second, the criteria and procedures for hospital staff appointment are likely to be precise and likely to require a high level of suitable credentials in a particular field, in such settings. Third, the ability and willingness of the staff to discipline itself will be greater. Fourth, the standards of medical care to the community at large served by the hospital will be higher where there is a very highly structured, self-disciplined hospital medical staff.

MONEY AND DIVISIVENESS

Having practiced for years in solo and in a two-doctor practice, and then having been involved in larger-scale group practice settings, it has been my experience that while there are many sources of interpersonal conflict and stress within groups of doctors who work together, of which Hunterdon is one prototype, the greatest source of conflict in our society is over money.

It has been interesting for me to note Dr. Henderson's comments. He referred to the major event of 1967: The development of an incentive program for the full-time specialist staff. Dr. Henderson concluded that equal income regardless of specialty (or work load) was not productive, and that financial incentive remains a strong motivation for productivity.

With regard to the second conclusion, George Bernard Shaw warned us a great many years ago. Financial incentive is, of course, a strong motivator for almost all of us—though surely not the only one. But in medical practice, as it has developed in the United States and Canada, there is no evidence whatever that full productivity per se, for equally busy doctors, in one field of practice is different than productivity in another field. And we know that the highest earning and busiest doctors often have very shoddy practices. So, we are not really talking about productivity at all but about irrationalities in the fee-for-service method of payment. Which takes us back to Dr. Henderson's first conclusion. Does he really mean that equal income regardless of specialty is not productive? I think what he means is that an inequitous fee-for-service system leads doctors to reject equal income even though they may in fact be equally productive and carry equal work loads.

While I appreciate the problem, I do not agree with the solutions that have been undertaken at Hunterdon. While I appreciate the fact that Hunterdon County's doctors did not invent the fee-for-service system, I think it is a great pity that you have enshrined it and that the specialists have over the years begun to succumb to the divisiveness inherent in that system. After all, the fee system was not handed down on Mount Sinai amidst thunder, lightning, and with burning bushes! For the first ten years there was a salary arrangement. This was then modified by an incentive system which has made some of the specialists far more equal than others. And yet, many reasonable persons would argue that it is good sense for doctors and others with equal training and equal lengths of experience, who work equal lengths of time, to get equal pay.

The fee schedules of the medical profession are not rational. These schedules, as my colleagues and I think we have shown in our Canadian studies, reflect the biases of a medicine preoccupied with surgical and other technical procedures. Seeing patients quickly and carrying out procedures is far more remunerative than talking, listening, counselling, planning, advising.

In our Canadian studies—and we do not believe findings in the United States would be much different—we found that the fee schedules permitted a radiologist to earn as much in 15 hours as did a family doctor in 45 hours. Likewise, the obstetrician-gynecologist and internist were able to earn twice as much per hour as did the family doctor, and the surgeon earned three times as much per hour—both in his office and in the hospital—as did the family doctor.

For Canada as a whole—and the situation is about the same in the United States—five surgical specialties are at the top of the income ranks for doctors' earnings while internal medicine, pediatrics, psychiatry, and family practice were at the bottom.

The fee system deals unequally with equals. It creates divisions between specialists and family doctors and, in Hunterdon as elsewhere, it has created divisiveness between specialists. Some argue that medical care prices, for various kinds of doctors' services, obey the market laws of supply and demand. But surely this is sheer rubbish. Market forces are *not* operative within the medical profession's fee system. Prices have been set unilaterally, are *not* negotiated with the consumer, and have *not* been revised over the years to equate length of training with time spent.

The highest priority, in my judgment, should be given to the Hunterdon Medical Center's returning to the original principles underlying remuneration of its medical staff: *equality*. Yes, there can be incentives, but not based on fee-related volume of work. A kickback of a percentage of fee earnings to an individual doctor is *not* an incentive for a group effort. It is a disincentive to the principles underlying your original efforts.

Further, I believe, from my own experiences in other rural and urban settings in both Canada and the United States, where it may be even more difficult to recruit specialists than it is in rural New Jersey, that it is quite possible to attract specialists who are willing to work on the basis of true pooling and sharing of skills, knowledge, and income, on an egalitarian basis. Of course, incentives are necessary. The base pay has to be satisfactory. Yours, quite frankly, seems not to be very satisfactory. And are the fringe benefits broad enough? And are the academic status and teaching opportunities that have been spelled out to date really attractive at present?

Also, and I know I am on sensitive turf here, do you need to re-examine the relation of the doctors to one another, to the center and to its board of trustees as an entity? Do the doctors see themselves as involved in decision-making concerning the center, or do they tend to see themselves as cogs in a somewhat impersonal machine?

Perhaps you are going to have to put greater efforts into redevelopment of your specialist staff, with a shift in focus. Perhaps you have begun to recruit doctors overly trained in the new sub-technologies in your small hospital, when what you need are specialists who will provide the ABCs of their special areas, and refer sub-specialty problems to larger centers. For example, the study by Drs. Trussell and Elinson showed that your population had a lot of visual problems and that many were not being cared for. A lot of people needed eyeglasses but didn't have them. Does your eye department have a county-wide screening program, on an ongoing basis, for eye defects and their correction? Similar questions can be asked in a number of other specialty areas.

You now have about 34 full-time specialists! The question I put to you is: How many are enough? Are you running the risk of overdoing specialization activities in your county, and at the same time still ignoring some of the core primary care, preventive care, home care, follow-up care, continuing care activities that are at the heart of good and sensitive health services? Are you really working to wed personal health care, preventive care, and public health activities in your county under the center's umbrella? And are your specialists really working primarily as consultants and as educators?

Perhaps you will need to expand your family practice department to include a major county-wide effort in community preventive medicine, dovetailed with a further redefinition of what specialists in your center will and will not do, and how they will relate more closely to meeting everyday unmet needs for health care in the county.

That leads me to make an aside to note that it would be fascinating to develop an evaluation strategy to look at where you've come from and where you're going. It seems to me that it would be rather simple to match a population along multiple parameters with characteristics similar to those of the

Hunterdon County population and to do, on a limited number of indicators, a study of unmet needs for care and services. I have a feeling that this county would come out a big winner and that such a demonstration could have very substantial national impact. Also, as a general evaluation strategy you could pick a number of indicators of sensitivity of your service and monitor such indicators on an ongoing basis.

THE NEXT TWO DECADES

You have begun a great experiment and I think you really have avoided a two-class system of care in your county. But in the next two decades, unless you deal with some of the questions I've tried to identify in my comments, I think you run the risk of going downhill. Now, some will argue that a breakup of the present set-up would be an advance, not a retreat. Why not, for example, have a more open situation—specialists and family doctors primarily on fees both in the hospital and in the community? Or, why not have a small group of full-time salaried specialists in the hospital and specialists in the community working on a traditional fee basis? Why not loosen the present very tightly structured medical staff organization? The answer, on an interim basis, lies in your accomplishments to date, or your apparent accomplishments. You've succeeded in having an adequate supply of specialists, as we understand ratios at the moment, who serve as consultants to the family doctors. The present arrangements do seem to have avoided the worst features of competition between specialists and family doctors. To open your system could lead to a less equitable supply of specialists and family doctors than you have at present. What you may need to assure your survival and expansion is a rededication to your original principles, not a retreat, and surely the development of a county-wide pre-payment mechanism tied to the principles of a health maintenance organization.

Quite frankly, I would, in the not too distant future, have

another go at the notion of all the specialists and all the family doctors becoming involved in such an arrangement.

ATYPICAL DEMONSTRATION OR REPLICATABLE

Accepting the fact that the Hunterdon Medical Center was created in a setting that was right for such a development, with informed lay leadership represented by really exceptional people like Mr. Wescott, and by exceptional professionals like Drs. Trussell and Pellegrino, still I hate to say, and cannot accept the fact, that what you have done is an atypical demonstration rather than representing a replicatable set of ideas and concepts that are needed in a great many counties throughout this broad land. But this can only come about if in the next two decades three major pieces of legislation are implemented on the national level in this country, and then applied by the states or on a regional basis. Because it seems to me that what is needed in this country is pressure towards a fundamental restructuring of both the financing and the organization of health care services.

The struggle for equitable health care for all Americans is going to take place in the context of the potential of three key enactments: the Health Maintenance Organization Bill, the Comprehensive Health Manpower Training Act and the Nurses Training Act, and national health insurance. In my judgment, every effort should be expended to rally support for the Kennedy-Mills national health insurance proposals. These would give you the tools in your county to help do the job you're already doing so well even better. Every pressure needs also to be exerted to assure that the manpower enactments lead to a recommitment to good primary health care and to family medical practice. It's sad to see that this thrust was started and then seemingly thwarted by present policies at the national level.

Finally, to assure the spread of the Hunterdon ideas and

concepts, the Health Maintenance Organization pre-paid group health center concept does need massive support tied to an educational program that will make such programs a truly available option. In this process, in my judgment, every effort must be exerted to chip away at the inequities of the fee-for-service system of medical practice and where possible to replace this system with other alternative ways to pay doctors.

I salute you, Hunterdon Medical Center, on this, your 20th anniversary! Please invite me back in 1993. And thank you for inviting me today.

MEDICAL EDUCATION AND THE
COMMUNITY HOSPITAL: THE LONG VIEW

•

Richard M. Magraw, M.D.

The involvement of community hospitals in medical education began with the rotating internship. This was traditionally less a formal part of education than a polishing off of clinical experience prior to entrance to practice. Some medical schools required it before awarding the MD degree; however, that requirement ceased altogether by the time of World War II. Since that start, community hospitals have become progressively more involved in specialty training or graduate medical education, and now more recently in undergraduate education. Hospital administration and boards of trustees have justified their involvement in the educational processes:

1. As an investment in improved quality of care of patients through stimulation of staff and the associated, more or less, unavoidable continuing education;

2. As a device for attracting professional staff to the institution and particularly professional staff of high quality; or

3. As a means of bringing into the community for possible recruitment a stream of medical students, interns and/or residents who are thereby "exposed" to the advantages of life in the community.

More recently, as hospital costs have continued to mount, interested individuals such as Pennsylvania's Herbert Dennenberg, have directly challenged these explanations or questioned the rationale for support of these programs out of patient care funds for the "cost effectiveness" of educational programs in relation to patient care.

I propose to analyze here what occurs when medical education programs are interwoven with the medical care system of a community and to describe how this process is taking place all over the country as old relationships are restructured between the process and the system of medical education and the system of medical care and particularly of the charity system of medical care. For some 50 years following the period of rapid change in American medical education, which was not so much introduced as it was documented by the 1910 publication of the Flexner Report, American medical education, per se, remained stable and with its basic character unchanging. Now that period of stability is at an end, and during the past eight or ten years the way medical students are taught has undergone sweeping revisions. (We need to make a distinction here between the changing process of medical students' education per se and the changes going on in and around the medical school itself or in the academic medical center.)

The interweaving between the system of medical education and the system of medical care which has been occurring is resulting not so much in new social arrangements as in the formation of new social institutions.

We are seeing a fading and, I believe, the passing of the predominant academic medical center of the past generation and the coming into being in its stead of an academic medical network or of a regional system of education in medicine and the so-called health sciences. The importance of medical education in the community hospital in this new circumstance is only now being recognized. That is to say, the importance of the community hospital in medical education is now being recognized in the university and the nearly essential role of medical education in the community hospital has only recently come to be recognized by the public. Before amplifying that assertion let me emphasize that in making it I do not wish to be understood as adding my voice to those who might defend the increasing costs of medical care and particularly of hospital services by laying an educational burden on the community hospital. Obviously, there must be careful allocation of costs between those resources which are used for patient care and those for education, and it is evident that we are in for a period of social and political negotiations over this point during which a kind of shell game is likely to be played by various interested parties. In these negotiations it will be important to clarify as precisely as possible the value of and demand for services in patient care, education, and research, which are jointly produced for somewhat different customers.

Returning now to the earlier point that the value of having medical education take place in the system of medical care of a community or region has only recently come to be understood, I would assert that the reason for recent pressures for establishing new medical schools in communities lacking them has been misunderstood or too simplistically understood as a drive to get more doctors. What has really been behind it, in my view, has been a not entirely clearly articulated but nonetheless widely held conviction that medical education is too important a process to be limited to the cities which already possess it and that localities that do not have it are disadvantaged. It has become the common experience of many regions in America having populations of a million or so that their medical care systems are unable to sustain or renew themselves without an inner framework—an endoskeleton of medical education. This was, for example, the situation in Illinois—a state with an 11.5 million population, 7 million in Chicago where there were six medical schools, and 4.5 million downstate where there were no medical schools. The insistence in Illinois was not so much to produce more medical students, per se, but to decentralize medical education. Later, as ideas became more refined, it was clear that people wanted a regionalized system of medical education.

I can put this in another perspective and make the important point that what medical education is or what medical schools do for society has changed progressively as society has changed by stating that in the past generation six new missions have been added to medical schools and in this process their nature, functions, and designations have been radically altered. I believe you all know the story. Thirty years ago, when I graduated, a medical school was pretty much defined by its name, i.e., a school for doctors and a school whose product was the graduate with an MD degree.

In the succeeding 10 to 15 years medical schools acquired four of their new missions. They became increasingly the places where the most advanced and specialized services were provided, i.e., they became medical centers of world-wide repute. Then they became graduate schools for training in clinical specialties. Then they became research institutes, and then centers of continuing education. Each of these was an added mission progressively changing the characteristics of the institutions and, in the process, their designation was gradually changed from medical college to medical center or to academic medical center. In the past ten years, in some instances, with the addition of yet another mission, that of providing a full spectrum of educational programs in the health sciences, the former medical school evolved further into a university of health sciences although the name academic health science center is generally used.

In the past few years still another mission or function has been added, namely that of medical education, serving as a framework or an endoskeleton to support the tissue of the medical care system for a region. The metaphor is not entirely apt since the patient care system is also supportive of education. A more apt figure is that of an interwoven fabric with strands of medical education interwoven with those of medical care.

Coming back to an analysis of the role of education in the community hospital, we should emphasize that the relationship between medical education and teaching and the promotion of high quality medical services in the community is not a simple one. Persons who insist, as I do, that educational programs in communities improve patient care in these communities have little proof for this assertion and may advance differing arguments to support their views. This variation in views as to the importance of medical education in promoting quality of care in a community is partly a function of the degree of sophistication about this. My own presentation is to propose an analogy between the kind of sophisticated analysis needed to understand the effects of education with Maimonides' eight stages of charity and the subtle distinctions and penetrating insights concerning the nature of charity which are embodied in that famous progression. You will recollect that Maimonides, recognizing that all acts of giving were not equally effective, once made a formal ranking of the eight stages of charity as follows:

Stage 1 Giving grudgingly.

Stage 2 Giving ungrudgingly but inadequately.

Stage 3 Giving on solicitation (that is, after having been asked).

Stage 4 Giving before being asked but with the gift and giving known to both giver and receiver.

Stage 5 Giving in which the giver is known to the recipient but the donor does not know to whom it goes.

Stage 6 Giving in which the recipient is known to the donor but the giver is unknown to the recipient (indeed, the fact of the gift may be unknown).

Stage 7 Giving without knowing to whom the gift is going and in such a way that the recipient does not know who has given.

Stage 8 Conducting one's own life in a way that takes away the occasion for charity and influencing society toward that end.

Although this progression of understanding about human needs and human kindness involves nuances and subtleties, the points made are profound and consequential. In a somewhat like manner, we can analyze the ways in which medical education in a community can affect the quality of personal health services provided there.

In this instance, the stages are not quite so crisp and neat. In the abstract it is possible to separate the different stages of understanding of medical education in the community hospital in relation to its effect on the quality of patient care in the community into some such categories as the following:

Stage 1   Concern with the symbols of an educational identity, e.g., for the individual physician the achievement of an academic appointment, or academic title, or for the hospital the achievement of a signed affiliation document, which denotes a teaching hospital.

Stage 2   Concern with courses and instructors. "We've got the franchise, let's buy some players and a ballpark and get into the league" expresses this rather superficial involvement.

Stage 3   Concern with instruction and with teaching per se, i.e., with teaching facilities, teaching equipment, and teaching paraphernalia of all kinds.

Stage 4   Concern with the students' learning per se, as opposed to instruction.

Stage 5   Concern with what is to be learned and the nature of the learning process.

Stage 6   Concern with development of a total clinical milieu of a quality which will enhance student learning, e.g., the hospital recognizes that only by becoming more excellent in the care its staff provides to patients can learning be improved.

Stage 7   Preoccupation with the assessment of

what has been learned and hence of the effectiveness of the learning process.

Stage 8   Perfection of feedback mechanisms from the needs of the community to defining goals and learning processes. There is an aphorism among educators to the effect that at first you teach more than you know, then you teach what you know, and ultimately you help students learn what is useful.

This progression suggests that becoming a real teaching hospital, i.e., an educational instrument which is reciprocally enriched by the educational programs carried out, is a gradual and progressive affair. It must be emphasized that while there is a substantial body of opinion among those who are experienced that their educational programs do, in fact, improve patient care, there is little actual proof of this.

The above progression is stated in highly abstract terms and does not define with any specificity the levels of commitment to medical education (and hence of effect on patient care) which are actually identifiable now, either among the medical staff members or in the hospitals themselves where any commitment is present. To provide a more concrete basis for discussion, here is another formulation of the varying levels or stages of involvement in or commitment to medical education which can be observed in hospitals.

I. MEDICAL EDUCATION AS AN INDIVIDUAL ACADEMIC PRETENSION

We have all observed how not uncommonly by dint of extraordinary effort (sometimes by weekly trips of a couple of hundred miles) occasional individual physicians will continue to serve in some capacity as a member of a medical faculty. At this level the individual medical staff member obtains and maintains an academic appointment in a medical school operating essentially on his own. (I use the term pretension not primarily in the sense of a claim or of mere ostentation but in the literal and derivative meaning of a stretching forth, i.e., an aspiration.)

The physician's medical school appointment is not at all related to his hospital staff membership or his medical role in the community but is a result of services at the (distant) medical school, for instance as a result of working as an instructor in the clinic. In the simplest case an individual physician seeks a faculty appointment (and may expend prodigious effort to get it) based primarily on his own accomplishments and professional qualifications rather than on a specific instructional assignment or performance. In short, the motivation to undertake this first stage may be less that of teaching and more that of wanting to be known as a faculty member. The process of student education can be almost incidental, with regard to motivation, to participate in educational programs. At this level the staff member often understands education as instruction. This is to say he usually operates in the apprenticeship mode and frame of reference and not infrequently participates in the student's education as a chore rather than as a personal learning opportunity and privilege.

The title may be important as an embellishment to the physician's identity as a practitioner. It may, for instance, assist him in the jockeying for position in the hospital staff pecking order and provide part of the credentials of recognized professional excellence. A clinical appointment is sought by some as the next accolade beyond board certification. This kind of educational involvement of the staff of a community hospital does not have anything like a maximal effect on patient care, but even if this is all there is to it, it is probably not without effect on the quality of care in the hospital and community because at the very least it keeps information channels with the academic medical center more open. Moreover, since people tend to live up to their pretensions, a clinical assistant professor of medicine tends to behave in certain desirable ways in his practice because he holds that title.

II. MEDICAL EDUCATION AS AN INSTITUTIONAL PRETENSION

Here the community hospital or medical center does not see itself as an educational institution but serves simply as the place wherein (nominal) medical education programs are located. Its own process of patient care may be largely untouched by any educational processes occurring on the premises. The hospital accepts (perhaps tolerates is a better word) and supports education as a necessary but essentially alien mission. Most often the "educational programs" are at the level of internships and residencies, although to an increasing extent the community hospital is a locus where some part of the clinical training of medical students is carried out.

At the level of residency training the training programs are often mere devices for obtaining services of well-paid, often foreign-trained house officers who, in many instances, receive haphazard instruction in their training as well.

At the undergraduate level the hospital's views of a medical school affiliation, often more prized as a way of getting a preferred listing in the Green Book (of accredited internships and residencies) than as a partnership geared to enhancing student learning, fall into two categories, both of which assume the educational programs are separate from the hospital and its missions.

(a) The first view is that the undergraduate educational program is a kind of medical school pearl in a hospital oyster. It adds luster, shows the organism off to glamorous advantage and enhances its market value but is essentially an inert foreign body,

and doesn't interfere with the metabolism of the
parent organism. It is both alien and inert in respect to the hospital.

(b) The second view is that while the educational mission may be alien in the hospital it is not inert. It
requires and is entitled to support and space of its
own and can with care be fitted into the interstices
of the existing structure like a piece into a jigsaw
puzzle without seriously disturbing existing arrangements or the hospital's basic mission of patient care. However, it may need to be trimmed to
size and boundaries must be carefully drawn and
territories meticulously observed.

It is not clear how much this level of commitment to
education by the hospital improves the quality of care in the
institution or the community. The effectiveness of those so-
called graduate medical educational programs wherein interns
and residents (usually foreign graduates) are recruited by a
hospital as "hired help" which the institution provides for its
medical staff in improving the quality of care is particularly
open to question. Even here there are often some beneficial
effects but over-all and in its ultimate effects I believe such
programs erode the quality of care which Americans receive
by importing poorly trained physicians. However, institutions, too, tend to live up to their pretensions and if a hospital
claims its internships and residencies are primarily educational
programs there are significant pressures to make them so.
Accrediting bodies have been under considerable pressure
from practitioners and hospitals not to exert really decisive
and controlling regulation of residency programs which exist
to provide a convenient service more than education. Correspondingly, the "exploitation" of foreign graduates, the
countries they came from, and the American public and the
erosion of quality of the American system of care continues
unchecked.

III. THE INDIVIDUAL PRACTITIONER OR HOSPITAL STAFF MEMBER MAKES A COMMITMENT TO PROVIDE MEDICAL EDUCATION IN HIS COMMUNITY HOSPITAL

Once the hospital has gotten involved in medical education it is up to the individual staff members to decide their own commitment. At the level of involvement described here the individual practitioner in some degree changes his personal identity or self-concept and becomes, in part, an instructor or professor in function whether he does or not in name.

He invests himself principally in relation to the structure of an academic department or an academic rank. He recognizes that the traditional channelized sequencing of a period of training and then life-long practice which was appropriate for a time when society and professional practice were more static than now is not adequate for current realities.

He recognizes that arduous as his initial education was, the task of staying educated while practicing is even more difficult. Correspondingly, he adapts his life style and creates a pattern of professional practice to accomplish this. Individual practitioners of this kind may effect the quality of care provided an entire area throughout their professional lifetimes.

IV. MEDICAL EDUCATION AS AN INSTITUTIONAL MISSION AND COMMITMENT

Here the hospital or medical center as a whole (i.e., the medical staff, administration, governing board acting together) accepts as fundamental to its style of operating a full participation in educational programs. The graduate and under-graduate programs are no longer foreign bodies in the tissues of the hospital. They are, in fact, no longer just the medical school's programs but become, to the hospital, "our" programs. In my experience, when this occurs the quality of medical care in the community is substantially better than it is elsewhere. It has come to be understood that good patient care is not merely related to medical education—it *is* medical education and vice versa. One of my more conservative academic colleagues, in an editorial in a leading medical journal, recently defined the university as "a compound (i.e., walled enclosure) for study and research." But neither research nor study are ever ends in themselves to be walled off from life and society. They are always means—means for helping real people in real situations. It is probable that the walled enclosure, the campus, will be decreasingly important in all higher education, not just medicine, in the coming generation The university, in any event, is not a campus but a state of mind.

The Renaissance concept of the university was not a geographical one but a philosophical one signifying the interplay among individual minds with reciprocal stimulation and enhanced productivity. For the benefit of patients today and tomorrow, the medical center and the hospital can be and should be such a place.

V. SYMBIOSIS BETWEEN THE MEDICAL CARE SYSTEM OF A REGION OR POPULATION AND THE MEDICAL EDUCATIONAL SYSTEM OF THAT REGION

This level of involvement or commitment has not yet fully come into being in many places in the country and even where it is in evidence it is not always recognized. At this level, medical education has as one of its accepted missions the support of the system of medical care and health services of the community or region. In turn, the medical educational programs are supported by the region.

In the past decade, many metropolitan areas and regional populations have become more aware that their hospitals and, indeed, their entire systems of medical care and health services cannot remain really first-class instruments of medical service unless they are integrally related to the full spectrum of medical educational activities. In a somewhat similar way, academic medical centers have been learning that they cannot flourish without integral relationships with the community. They require continuous feedback mechanisms regarding their effectiveness and the appropriateness of personnel trained in relation to the shifting medical care and health service needs of the population. Faculties of such centers have three major obligations: One, to determine what is to be learned; two, to develop arrangements which permit and facilitate the student learning that which is to be learned; three, to ascertain whether these things were in fact learned. Of these, perhaps the most important is the first.

In short, the system of medical education and the system of medical care are increasingly interwoven. Neither can flourish without the other. The community hospital's involvement in and commitment to medical education must be understood as part of the involvement of the entire system of health services in programs for education in the health sciences.

In order that patients of the next year and next decade should be properly served, medical education today needs to be an integral part of the medical care system. The effects on patient care ten years from now of having medical education today related to community needs through community hospitals will be substantial. The absence of such influence today will materially diminish the quality of medical care services a decade from now.

THE HOSPITAL'S RESPONSIBILITY FOR COMMUNITY HEALTH SERVICES

•

Anne Ramsay Somers

This paper deals with the fourth concept in the complex of imaginative ideas and pragmatic developments that has come to be known as the "Hunterdon model." As stated in the symposium program, this concept provides "that the community hospital should assume responsibility for, and serve as a focus for, the provision of a wide spectrum of health care services." Ideally, it aims at assuring access to all aspects of personal health care—from health education and primary care at one end of the comprehensive care spectrum to post-hospital rehabilitation and long-term care at the other end.

In the time available to me, I shall try to do four things:

1. Identify the minimum requirements for implementation of the concept;

2. Appraise the extent to which the concept is, or is not, being generally adopted in the United States;

3. Identify the major obstacles preventing wider adoption; and

4. Hazard a guess as to the future.

THE BASIC CONCEPT

As one reviews the Hunterdon experience and explores the possibility for adoption or adaptation elsewhere, three requirements emerge as the *sine qua non* for success:

1. The hospital must be willing to commit a substantial portion of its professional, administrative, financial, and other resources to health care modalities other than the traditional in-patient services. This does not mean that all such services should be provided in the hospital itself. On the contrary, many can be better provided in other locations and by other institutions. But all such institutions, and all professionals involved in the process, should be affiliated or associated with the core hospital in such a way that the patient can be referred from one level of care to another without duplication of tests, records, or costs, and with the assurance of over-all quality and cost controls.

For the average community hospital this would probably mean provision of most secondary and some primary care on its own premises, affiliation with a medical school or major teaching hospital for most tertiary care, and supervision of additional primary and long-term care through affiliated institutions and professionals.

Hunterdon—with its balance of in-patient and ambulatory facilities, its strong emphasis on primary care, its three satellite family health centers, its continuing care facility, its community mental health center, home care program, methadone and alcoholism clinics, child evaluation center, its long-standing affiliations with medical schools and tertiary care centers, and its general assumption of responsibility for most components of the comprehensive care spectrum for the population of an entire county—comes closer to fulfilling this requirement than any other I know.

2. In order to develop and to operate the network of community health services contemplated in the first point, the core hospital must gradually transform itself into a community-wide "management system" with authority commensurate to its responsibility. The authority may be either *de facto*, as at Hunterdon, or *de jure*, if necessary.

The definition of "community" may be on the basis of geographical or socio-economic considerations or through explicit membership. At Hunterdon, the definition is related to county lines. As the only hospital in the county, the problem is far simpler than it would be in a multi-hospital community.

3. In order to acquire the authority and develop the "management system" contemplated in the second point, the leadership of the core hospital must be strong, cohesive, and acceptable to—preferably representative of—all major provider and consumer elements within the institution and within the community. The leadership must be able to unite these diverse elements in agreement on a common institutional goal: the assurance of high quality comprehensive health care to the defined population at a feasible price.

Although the Hunterdon leadership has been rebuffed on some issues—for example, its advocacy of an HMO-type financing mechanism—it has obviously been able to exercise effective authority and to implement the basic concept. The leadership—both lay and professional—has also been marked by an exceptionally high degree of public spirit and altruism (one might almost use the fast-vanishing term *noblesse oblige*) as well as competence.

The question inevitably arises whether this quality along with the *de facto* definition of community—the county—can be generally replicated, or whether some more formal method of assuring these two prerequisites is generally necessary.

CURRENT DIFFUSION OF THE CONCEPT

The Hunterdon concept has not only proved professionally and politically acceptable to the great majority of providers and consumers in Hunterdon County, it is also financially viable. There is evidence that good comprehensive health care is available to the residents of this county at lower costs than the state or national averages.

In this day of widespread concern for the rising costs of

health care, for the fragmentation of care, and the alleged irresponsibility of some health professionals and institutions, the Hunterdon model might seem an answer to the public's prayer. Has this been the case? How widely has the concept of hospital responsibility for a broad spectrum of health care been accepted and implemented?

Here, in New Jersey, some eight or ten of our stronger hospitals are moving—at varying rates of speed and with varying success—in this general direction. On the national scene, one thinks immediately of individual institutions— Massachusetts General in Boston, Mt. Sinai in New York City, Rush-Presbyterian-St. Luke's in Chicago, Mt. Zion in San Francisco, for example—that have struggled mightily to establish good ambulatory services, neighborhood health centers, community mental health centers, nursing homes, etc. Throughout the entire country one now hears a great deal of talk about the hospital as a "community health center." Many institutions have changed their names to reflect this new orientation.

The American Hospital Association is concerned with its leadership role in the entire health care field. The report of the Perloff Committee*, of which Lloyd Wescott was one of the most influential members, with its recommendation for the establishment of health care corporations, was a quantum leap forward in AHA thinking in this area. The health care corporation concept—at least partly based on the Hunterdon model—was brought to the attention of Congress and the general public through incorporation into the national health insurance bill sponsored by the AHA and introduced in 1972 by Congressman Ullman.

However, it is easy to be misled by individual examples and by general rhetoric. What *is* actually happening through-

* Special Committee on the Provision of Health Services of the American Hospital Association. The report was delivered in November 1970.

out the country? Is the *average* community hospital moving in this direction or not?

There is no definitive way of answering these questions. The data is incomplete, sometimes inconsistent, and even misleading. Nevertheless, an indication of trends can be obtained through analysis of the AHA data with respect to hospital services, published each year, formerly in the *Guide Issue*, now in the accompanying volume, *Hospital Statistics*.

Table 1 shows the comparative changes in the proportion of all United States community hospitals reporting selected services from 1962 to 1972. These are some of the more significant findings:

1. The percentage of hospitals with general intensive care units rose from 15 to 59 percent. In addition, by 1972, 35 percent had special cardiac intensive care facilities. In 1962, there was not even a category for open heart surgery. In 1972, 8 percent had open heart units.

2. Radioactive isotope facilities and electroencephalography—illustrative of the highly specialized, technologically sophisticated and capital-intensive services—increased from 25 percent to 66 percent and from 17 to 36 percent respectively.

3. Of the non-technological outreach services, the two which showed the most significant increases were psychiatric out-patient departments (in 1972 this included day care, night care, and other partial hospitalization programs), not reported in 1962, and 19 percent in 1972, and social service departments, rising from 15 to 41 percent.

4. Home care, a program strongly pushed by Medicare, Medicaid, and Blue Cross, rose from 4 percent of all community hospitals in 1962 to 7 percent in 1967, then declined again to 6 percent in 1972.

5. There was a modest rise in the proportion of hos-

TABLE 1

SELECTED SERVICES PROVIDED BY UNITED
STATES COMMUNITY HOSPITALS, 1962–1972[1]

	1962	1972
Number of hospitals reporting	5,395	5,456
	(%)	(%)
Intensive care unit–general	15.1	58.5
Intensive care–cardiac only	——	35.3
Open heart surgery	——	8.2
Radioactive isotope facility[2]	24.8	66.4
Electroencephalography	16.9	36.3
Self-care unit	——	3.9
Extended care unit	——	11.3
Rehabilitation services[3]	6.5	11.8
Psychiatric out-patient[4]	——	19.2
Out-patient department	40.8	27.5
Emergency room	93.6	86.6
Social service department	15.1	40.5
Family planning	——	6.4
Genetic counselling	——	2.8
Home care	3.8	6.2

[1] Non-Federal, short-term general, and other special hospitals.
[2] 1972 includes both diagnostic and therapeutic units.
[3] 1972 includes in- and out-patient units.
[4] 1972 includes partial hospitalization programs.

Sources: For 1962: American Hospital Association, *Guide Issue,* August 1, 1963, Table 5, pp. 478–81. For 1972: AHA, *Hospital Statistics 1972,* Table 13-A, pp. 205–11.

pitals with rehabilitation units but, even in 1972, less than 12 percent had such services. Four services: self-help and extended care units, family planning, and genetic counseling—nonexistent in 1962—were reported by small proportions of hospitals in 1972.

6. Perhaps most surprising of all is the decline in hospitals with out-patient departments and even emergency rooms. While the small relative drop in emergency rooms may reflect some sensible consolidations or division of labor between nearby institutions, the much larger decline for out-patient departments is harder to explain. The latter drop is all the more striking if compared with the 1967 figure of 52 percent.

This may come as a surprise to those who have been watching the historic rise in out-patient visits. Those hospitals with OPDs *are* obviously experiencing a continuing dramatic rise in utilization. This may be precisely the reason that some hospitals closed these units while others are reluctant to take them on.

In the effort to probe some of the factors behind these broad over-all trends, the same 15 services have been broken down according to hospital ownership, size, and geographical region (Tables 2 and 3).

Analyzed in terms of ownership, these are the principal trends:

1. The proprietaries are deeply involved in most of the technological services. By contrast, they show the least commitment to the various humanistic and outreach programs.

2. The voluntaries are the obvious pace-setters for the industry with respect to both technological and humanistic services. In both areas, their commitment is greater than for either of the other categories. Yet

TABLE 2

SELECTED SERVICES PROVIDED BY UNITED STATES HOSPITALS[1] BY OWNERSHIP AND SIZE 1962–1972

(percent of reporting hospitals)

| | BY OWNERSHIP | | | | | | BY SIZE | | | | | |
| | 1962 | | | 1972 | | | 1962 | | | 1972 | | |
	Vol.	*Profit*	*Gov't.*	*Vol.*	*Profit*	*Gov't.*	*100–199*	*300–399*	*500+*	*100–199*	*300–399*	*500+*
Intensive care	17.7	9.1	12.3	68.1	45.6	44.2	15.2	46.0	64.0	77.2	97.8	97.6
Intensive cardiac	——	——	——	41.4	20.1	28.6	——	——	——	33.3	64.8	88.6
Open heart	——	——	——	11.2	0.8	5.1	——	——	——	3.3	23.8	66.9
Radioactive iso.[2]	32.4	8.4	15.7	84.7	43.0	38.6	36.1	86.0	95.7	73.0	169.6	188.2
Electroencephal.	21.5	7.8	11.0	45.1	32.5	20.3	16.3	65.6	95.0	40.7	91.9	98.0
Self-care	——	——	——	5.3	0.5	2.3	——	——	——	3.6	11.7	16.8
Extended care	——	——	——	12.1	1.5	13.4	——	——	——	13.4	12.7	13.2
Rehab. [3]	8.0	0.9	6.0	15.0	1.7	9.2	5.2	21.6	52.0	7.1	33.1	81.9
Psychiatric [4]	——	——	——	22.0	5.2	19.3	——	——	——	14.5	48.1	91.8
Out-patient	41.6	43.1	37.3	33.0	15.7	21.1	34.4	76.8	93.5	22.1	57.4	86.2
E. R.	93.8	88.6	96.2	89.0	68.5	88.6	96.6	99.2	99.3	91.1	97.8	99.6
Social service	18.6	2.0	14.5	50.6	22.4	27.3	14.5	58.4	85.6	49.8	83.6	93.7
Family planning	——	——	——	7.4	1.0	6.3	——	——	——	2.9	16.7	38.2
Genetic counsel.	——	——	——	3.2	——	3.1	——	——	——	1.5	5.2	24.8
Home care	4.1	2.5	3.8	8.5	1.0	3.4	2.9	14.4	23.7	7.4	11.7	23.4

[1] Non-Federal, short-term general, and other special hospitals.

[2] 1972 includes both diagnostic and therapeutic units.

[3] 1972 includes in- and out-patient units.

[4] 1972 includes partial hospitalization programs.

Sources: For 1962: American Hospital Association, *Guide Issue*, August 1, 1963, Table 5, pp. 478–81.
For 1972: AHA, *Hospital Statistics 1972*, Table 13-A, pp. 205–11.

TABLE 3

SELECTED SERVICES PROVIDED BY ALL UNITED STATES HOSPITALS, BY REGION, 1973

(percent of reporting hospitals)

	N.E.	Mid-Atlantic	So. Atlantic	East N.C.	East S.C.	West N.C.	West S.C.	Mountain	Pacific
Intensive care	54.6	64.0	50.9	57.2	40.4	44.3	43.5	51.3	65.8
Intensive cardiac	27.9	36.2	34.1	31.8	27.8	29.2	24.6	29.4	34.9
Open heart	6.2	9.7	5.3	9.0	5.5	4.9	7.3	7.8	9.2
Radioactive iso. [1]	62.6	86.4	59.8	70.9	42.3	38.9	42.3	42.6	68.6
Electroencephal.	46.7	53.4	35.6	44.7	24.3	26.3	28.0	26.1	46.7
Self-care	6.9	6.8	7.5	7.0	3.9	3.8	2.2	3.3	2.9
Extended care	12.1	13.9	7.5	12.7	13.9	18.9	3.8	16.7	16.2
Rehab. [2]	23.8	27.9	11.7	17.0	4.4	11.8	6.8	12.7	17.1
Psychiatric [3]	47.0	44.7	27.3	28.3	17.9	22.1	15.4	25.5	31.5
Out-patient	45.1	49.1	28.5	30.9	20.6	23.2	20.2	32.5	31.5
E. R.	66.4	74.7	73.3	76.4	78.8	79.5	75.8	81.6	75.2
Social service	74.9	78.7	45.6	54.8	38.4	33.4	24.2	35.5	48.5
Family planning	12.8	15.9	8.1	6.3	4.5	4.8	4.2	9.6	8.2
Genetic counsel.	2.8	5.9	2.8	3.0	1.4	1.9	1.2	1.6	4.4
Home care	11.0	15.1	4.4	5.4	4.5	5.3	1.0	6.6	6.4

[1] 1972 includes both diagnostic and therapeutic units.

[2] 1972 includes in- and out-patient units.

[3] 1972 includes partial hospitalization programs.

Sources: AHA, *Hospital Statistics 1972*, Table 13-B, pp. 212–218.

with respect to home care, family planning, and extended care, the proportion of hospitals involved ranges downward from 15 percent. Only a third have organized out-patient departments.

In terms of size, it is not surprising that the larger hospitals have the stronger technological programs. However, the variation in humanistic and outreach programs is more striking than might have been anticipated. Lack of adequate resources—both financial and manpower—can explain the fact that only a third of the hospitals in the 100–199 bed range have a cardiac intensive care unit. But why do only 7 percent have a rehabilitation unit?

The general heavy emphasis on technological services and relatively poor showing for ambulatory and outreach programs is a nation-wide phenomenon. However, there are some significant regional variations. For example, 17 percent of the Mountain States hospitals have extended care units; only 4 percent of those in the adjoining West South Central region.

Hospitals in the Mid-Atlantic region are consistently stronger with respect to the outreach services, especially when contrasted with the South. Nearly 80 percent of the Mid-Atlantic group have social service departments; only 24 percent in the West South Central area. Nearly half of the Mid-Atlantic group have OPDs; only about 20 percent in the two Southern Central regions. Home care units range from 15 percent in the Mid-Atlantic down to 1 percent in the West South Central.

I do not claim too much for these "quick and dirty" figures. But despite the crudeness of the methodology as well as the data, the figures are of such an order of magnitude that it is impossible not to conclude that the average hospital of the early 1970s remains pretty much what it was a decade ago—a citadel of specialized, technologically-oriented inpatient care. Efforts to broaden the spectrum to include ambulatory care, preventive care, psychiatric care, rehabilitation, social services, and extended care have made some im-

pact, especially in the larger hospitals in the Mid-Atlantic—
and to a lesser extent the Pacific—states. In most of the
country, however, most conspicuously in the South, such
services are few and far between.

The facts are thus quite different from the rhetoric. Some
students of the health care scene, including myself, have been
so eager to see the hospital espouse this broader role along the
lines of the Hunterdon concept that we may have engaged
in some wishful thinking. Hunterdon, in 1973, is not as unusual as it was in 1953 but, in this respect at least, the Hunterdon concept remains distinctly a minority pattern.

MAJOR OBSTACLES TO DIFFUSION
OF THE CONCEPT

Why should this be so? Why, if the idea of the hospital as
community health center is so attractive, the viability of the
idea demonstrated, and a number of our most progressive
hospitals moving in this direction, why has there been so little
over-all movement and, in some respects, even a clear retro-
gression?

The complete answer, of course, is highly complex and
beyond the scope of this paper. It may be worthwhile, however, to point to a few of the major factors. They are not
listed in any order of priority. I tried to do this but gave up.
The hen-and-egg syndrome is obvious.

1. *Medical staff opposition or at least indifference to hospital involvement in primary and/or long-term care.* This
attitude is understandable. Most hospital staffs are dominated
by surgeons or other physicians whose professional lives have
been centered on acute, largely in-patient, care. The patients
they see every day, the problems they encounter, are in this
category. Most are aware of the pressing need for better
primary and long-term care but feel it is not their responsibility and fear that greater hospital involvement in such

modalities will result in diminution of resources available for their own work. Their fears are, of course, partly justified.

In any case, this point of view is still dominant in many—probably most—hospitals, whether or not the medical staff is officially represented on the board of trustees. It is unlikely to change in the near future, short of some strong external pressure.

2. *The financial bias toward in-patient care still inherent in most existing health insurance.* The professional bias toward in-patient care is strongly reinforced, from the point of view of hospital management, by the fact that the typical health insurance policy is also strongly skewed in this direction.

Despite years of effort to change this on the part of health care authorities and a few of the more progressive carriers, including Blue Cross and Prudential, very little progress has been made. Even Medicare, whose architects and administrators are fully aware of the distortion resulting from over-emphasis on in-patient care, contains some of the same bias—especially with respect to preventive health services.

Nowhere is the circular relationship between cause and effect clearer. For example, lack of third-party reimbursement is widely and convincingly cited as one reason for failure to develop more effective home care programs. Yet when home care was made available, on a limited basis, under Medicare and Medicaid, both doctors and patients apparently found it difficult to adjust their thinking and habits to the new circumstances. The 1967–1972 decline in proportion of hospitals with home care programs, already noted, was accompanied by a decline in the proportion of Medicare funds going for this purpose: the tragedy of self-fulfilling prophecy.

Why is it that the carriers find it so difficult to cover ambulatory care? The two reasons most frequently cited are: (a) inability to monitor utilization and to control abuse in non-institutional settings, and (b) the preference of most purchasers. Whatever the validity of this reasoning, the fact remains that we have been unable to establish governmental benefit standards which could have made ambulatory and other out-patient coverage mandatory. It is doubtful if any large-scale reform in this area is possible without some such standards.

3. *The difficult cost bind in which most hospitals now find themselves.* The hospitals have been crying "Wolf!" over their financial plight for so many years that it is difficult to be sure that the present situation is different from the virtually permanent crisis of the past two decades. There is reason to believe, however, that the situation is now more serious than at any time in the recent past—at least for many of our key urban hospitals, both public and voluntary.

For one thing, hospital costs are now so high that the slightest diminution in revenue can create an immediate credit or payroll crisis. Second, the various forces moving toward stricter control over hospital rates and reimbursement—state insurance commissioners, the Federal Economic Stabilization Program, Blue Cross, prospective rate-setting, etc.—are beginning to have real impact and the hospital's ability to pass on its rising costs to third party payers and taxpayers is increasingly limited.

As a result, the average hospital's maneuverability and its ability to experiment with innovative programs are even less than a few years ago. Unfortunately, the first programs to suffer are usually the new ambulatory and outreach programs. Not only are they generally less popular with the medical staff but, in the first years at least, they are often financial liabilities.

4. *The general passion for autonomy.* America is a country of strong individualists and this is a trait that applies to most of our institutions as well. The individualism of most physicians is legendary. The concept of the hospital as a management system inevitably involves surrender of some autonomy on the part of affiliated professionals and institutions. Resistance is understandable. Even the core hospital, which

would be operating the management system, fears the implications, possibly with some justification. Certainly, if an institution is to be given a legal franchise to operate such a system for a defined population group—as contemplated under the frequently discussed Ullman Bill, for example—it will, in turn, have to be accountable to some higher public authority.

Advocates of this approach say it is the best way to avoid far more stringent controls. But there are still many hospitals and physicians who believe that all controls can be avoided if they resist firmly enough. Even those who have advocated moderate state or non-governmental controls, as an alternative to rigid Federal regulation, frequently feel themselves betrayed by inept administration. The mood today in the industry appears to be one of increasing resistance to planning as well as regulation, rather than increasing accommodation. The outlook for any new program which might encumber the hospital in its effort to preserve its cherished autonomy is not encouraging.

5. The technological mystique as a reinforcement of the disappearing medical mystique. The layman's historical awe of the "medical mystique" has diminished during the past few decades with rising public educational and income levels and increasing emphasis on patient education rather than simple manipulation. The newer "technological mystique," or "technological fix" as it is sometimes called, has served to reinforce some of the old myths and strengthen conservative forces among both providers and consumers.

Ask the average man-on-the-street which is more important to make sure he doesn't die of a heart attack: (a) free and easy access to all the modern technology of cardiac resuscitation and heart surgery, or (b) his own diet, exercise, and life style. The majority will probably say the former. Hospital trustees, administrators, business and labor officials who choose the health insurance benefits for millions: the majority in all these lay groups are also strongly bemused by the miracles of modern medical technology and, when the crunch comes, are likely to give it higher priority than primary care or patient education. In this atmosphere, it is hardly surprising—although I find it distressing—that nearly ten times as many community hospitals have chosen to invest in a radioactive isotope facility rather than in a home care program. It will take more than exhortation to change this bias.

6. *A totally inconsistent and ineffective health policy.* Flexibility and pragmatic reaction on the part of government to changing needs are essential. But the 180 degree vacillations of the past few years have not only crippled most of the responsible governmental agencies but have made it extremely difficult for private bodies, including hospitals, to develop and sustain any coherent policy, other than survival and maintenance of the status quo.

Does the Federal government want to encourage HMOs or doesn't it? Does it want to encourage state regulation or doesn't it? Does it want a strong, effective private health insurance industry or doesn't it? Does it really want to make Medicare more efficient or not? Does it want hospitals to develop outreach or doesn't it?

On all of these and virtually every other issue of importance to the health care field, the present Administration has pursued a policy of such inconsistency, expediency, and lack of programmatic integrity that one is tempted to conclude that the primary aim was demoralization of the entire industry. I know this was *not* the aim. If it had been deliberate policy, it probably would not have succeeded so well!

If I single out the Federal government for special criticism in this respect, it's only because—having greater resources at its disposal—we have a right to expect more creative leadership from it. However, I don't mean to let the states off scot-free. When it comes to Medicaid, the certificate of need, and other areas within their jurisdiction, the record of most states has been almost as inconsistent as that of the Federal government.

WHAT OF THE FUTURE?

In view of the many formidable and not-easy-to-correct obstacles, I see little cause for optimism that the fourth Hunterdon concept—the hospital's assumption of responsibility for a broad spectrum of community health services— will be generally adopted in the foreseeable future. I hope I am mistaken. But for those who have been looking to this model as the method of choice for rationalization and regulation of the delivery system, the outlook is not encouraging.

When then? It seems to me there are three general routes we can travel or, more likely, a confused combination of the three:

1. Repudiation of all planning, as well as regulation, and an effort to force, or even impose, a free market and price competition on the health services industry;

2. Across-the-board Federal regulation, with or without some delegation of controls to regional or local "authorities";

3. Establishment of the Hunterdon health center concept by statute, probably in the form of a state franchise to hospitals willing and able to take on the responsibility.

A full exploration of each of these approaches would require a volume or more. All I can do here is suggest a few major implications under each of these headings and then pray that everyone will give serious study to these issues which are so portentous to the future of health care in the United States.

1. The free market concept has attracted many people, including some influential economists and government officials, who feel that the hospital—especially the voluntary hospital—has been overprotected from normal competition and more efficient would-be entrants into the health care marketplace. This view opposes any planning with teeth or regulation, and at least some of its advocates favor repealing the certificate-of-need laws.

A related view—not always held by the same people—opposes health insurance coverage of primary or routine care and would restrict benefits to costs of catastrophic proportions. The Administration's proposal to increase deductibles and coinsurance on Medicare beneficiaries is a tentative step in this direction. The aim, of course, is to force price competition by providers and greater restraint in the use of health services by consumers.

Some physicians and hospital officials, confused and angered by the current maze of regulations, are also attracted by this approach which, superficially at least, appears consistent with their concern for complete autonomy.

The attractions are obvious but the concept of a completely free market in health care will not stand up—either practically or philosophically. As a practical matter, the millions of Americans who now have something approaching first-dollar coverage for hospital care will not give it up. If the attempt is made to force price competition by high deductibles and coinsurance, people will simply buy additional complementary coverage as they have with Medicare. If the effort is made to make such first-dollar coverage illegal, as has been occasionally proposed, it will probably be declared unconstitutional.

If, on the other hand, the effort is made to force price competition on the providers while permitting the consumer to have first-dollar coverage, the competition cannot be meaningful. To the extent that it does work, the primary loser will be the good voluntary hospital that is trying to meet community needs, in education as well as care, and that is trying to provide its professionals with an attractive setting for work. The primary beneficiary will be the cut-rate proprietary institution, the free-standing "surgicenter," or the voluntary hospital that is a community hospital in name only, whose primary concerns are holding down costs, regardless of quality, and maximizing revenue-producing services, regardless of appropriateness.

Given the nation's admittedly excessive investment in high-cost hospital facilities, which neither the professions nor the public are prepared to see go down the drain, the net result of this futile effort will, almost certainly, be even higher costs than we have now plus even greater fragmentation and greater emphasis on high-cost revenue producing services, along with almost total neglect of primary care and the outreach services which the Hunterdon concept has demonstrated are not only desirable but feasible.

2. Across-the-board Federal regulation also has great superficial attraction to many. The idea of setting the stage for complete rationalization of the industry, through one stroke of a presidential pen, is obviously appealing to many who despair of voluntary or state initiatives. The Kennedy health security program is the clearest example of this approach but, far more likely, and just as ominous for the future, is the gradual consolidation of economic controls over the industry under the Economic Stabilization Program.

Where this will end no one knows. But with the Federal government already spending over $25 billion a year for health care, which puts health into primary competition with defense for the increasingly limited Federal dollar, it seems highly unlikely that the Administration will relinquish direct controls short of impressive demonstration of some effective alternative. Indeed, it seems possible that the industry could end up with the worst of both worlds: statutory "ceilings" on prices without any "floors"—i.e., no protection against cut-rate competition!

A variation on this theme would be to go the route of the regional authority. Congressman Roy is among those reportedly preparing legislation along this line. While this effort aims to assure decentralized decision-making and preservation of private health care, the net result could well be ineffectiveness—even worse than Comprehensive Health Planning and the Regional Medical Programs—or *de facto* Federal control.

One such proposal provides that the Department of Health, Education, and Welfare would establish the regions and approve, fund, and certify performance of the authorities. While an attempt is made to promote coordination with PSROs, it is more likely that the built-in conflicts would force eventual Federal take-over of both operations.

3. The idea of making the Hunterdon concept mandatory, of imposing responsibility for community health services on the voluntary hospital—by means of a legal franchise —may seem to many not only unattractive but almost a contradiction in terms. I suspect that some of the Hunterdon architects of the concept may feel that way. The genius of the idea may indeed be related to the voluntary pragmatic nature of its evolution.

But we are faced with rather a desperate situation in the industry. It is not that the individual consumer is so desperately concerned. The polls clearly indicate that he is not. But the reason he is not is because such a large proportion of the cost has been transferred to government and other third parties. These are the groups that are now left holding the bag and, unlike the individual consumer, they—particularly the Federal government—are in a position to take extreme, even punitive measures, against both the industry and consumers. Pressure is obviously building up in this direction. I can think of only one way to effectively head off such pressure. That is by the industry and the public—working at the state and community levels—fashioning some instrument for effective regulation short of direct Federal controls.

Is this likely to happen? The hospital officials and other health care experts reading this probably know better than I. I am not overly sanguine.

But I am sure of one thing. If it does happen, if we manage to put together some sort of pragmatic regulatory mechanism which can guarantee consumers access to high-quality comprehensive health care at a feasible price, without selling our souls to the Federal government, the Hunterdon model will be part of the solution. If we fail, if the Hunterdon model is lost in the morass of regulations and counter-regulations coming out of Washington and a thousand regional, state, and area offices throughout the country, those of us who have watched it evolve, who have been privileged to observe this tremendously impressive experiment, will look back on Hunterdon as a sort of medical Camelot—an island of humanism, altruism, and pragmatic creativity in a world overly preoccupied with technology, maximizing income, and theoretical solutions to human problems.

I don't mean to end on a completely pessimistic note. Particular Camelots and Utopias may pass but the search for alleviation of human disease and suffering will not cease; nor will the search for the perfectability of institutions and individuals to minister to these needs. In this ongoing quest, this journey whose end none of us can see, history will record that the Hunterdon experiment and the Hunterdon concept of the hospital as the central responsible focus of community health services have already made an admirable contribution.

HEALTH SERVICE FOR THE PUBLIC GOOD

•

John Schoff Millis

I have had the opportunity to learn about and see the Hunterdon Medical Center from time to time and have come to know some of the people who have been associated with the institution over the last 20 years. Therefore, I can—as a real outlander to this community and to this institution—offer on behalf of the country as a whole, and particularly those of us who are interested in medical affairs, our congratulations to an institution which has done much in a very brief period of time. You have every reason as a community, as a board of trustees, as members of the staff, as patients, to be extremely proud of what has been accomplished.

What I wish to do here is to state what I think were three decisions made some 20 to 25 years ago and to describe them in the context of the early days of the medical center, in the context of what has happened over a period of two decades, and then, lastly, to try to apply those basic decisions, which have become principles and central concepts, as one looks at the present and the future.

I chose the title "Health Service for the Public Good" because I think it describes better than any other simple set of words or phrases what I sensed about the Hunterdon record; it has been a health service of the community—that is, for the general welfare and the public good.

The three decisions which I believe were central in the initial days of the medical center, and which I wish to deal with here, are:

First, the purpose of the effort, of the commitment, was to design a health facility for *this* community—not a health facility for the State of New Jersey, or the United States of America, or for the world, but specifically for the community known as Hunterdon County. It began, therefore, not in dicta as what should be, but rather by the asking of questions about the needs and how they could be met. The first step really was that of Dr. Corwin and his associates who prepared that very interesting report which I have read again quite recently. It began essentially with the determination of the epidemiology of Hunterdon County, that is, what diseases and conditions affect Hunterdon County residents, what are their health problems? It was a report of the sources from which the residents of the county received their health care, an inventory of the health service resources—physicians, nurses, and other health professionals, clinics, hospitals, etc.

The second of the three decisions or principles is that if one is to design a health facility for *this* county and *this* community, it would then require the wholehearted participation of the community. Participation in planning, participation in financing, and most importantly it would require the caliber of leadership from, of, and on behalf of the community that this medical center has had. It has had, in my observation, perhaps the most remarkable leadership of any similar venture, and I am sure I also speak the gratitude of those whom this leadership has helped and assisted.

This second idea was to produce change, not by revolution, or—as we used to say in Vermont—by throwing the baby out with the bath water. Rather, it was to take that which was present, develop it, expand it, strengthen it, support it, and grow methodically step by step with the capacity to adjust with a changing environment and changing conditions and desires. This is encapsulated to me in the word evolution. It therefore began with the medical profession as it was then practicing in this community. It created a hospital with a concept of an open staff—that is, available for the practice of every physician in the community. It worked out a remarkable relationship to the public authority so that the usual separation, which is denoted by the terms public health on the one hand and private institution on the other, has never been a problem in this community.

The third basic decision was to include in the concept of a medical center the element of education. This, of course, to me as a person who has spent his life in higher education, is most gratifying. It signifies the recognition that learning is extremely important; that the opportunity to teach is also the opportunity to learn. Since a physician's life is a lifetime of learning, he needs the opportunity to teach, and he requires the stimulation and the energy which is provided by students.

In deciding to engage in some form of education you recognized the fact that you need manpower—physicians, nurses, social workers, health aides of many kinds, and that you cannot be totally dependent upon other people for the provision of that manpower, and, hence, must carry your share in the preparation of those who will provide health services in the future.

Now I wish to apply those three ideas, those three dicta, to what has happened in the 20 years since this institution was founded. It is very interesting to me that—this being the 20th anniversary—it means you have selected the year 1953, at least as the initial year of service, if not the initial year of the idea. It is almost the exact time which, when the history of health services in the 20th century is written, will be given a tremendous amount of attention by the historians. It was in the region of 1953 and 1954 that something rather phenomenal occurred in this country and throughout the world in every industrially developed nation. It was in those years that mortality rates, which had been declining year after year for the first half of the century (actually beginning in the latter part of the 19th century) bottomed out. It was at this time that life expectancy, which had been rising more than six months every year for the first half of the 20th century, suddenly stopped rising. Life expectancy has not increased significantly in the United States in the last 20 years. A very dramatic phenomenon, and I remind you that it was not only the United States in which it occurred but in every industrialized nation in the world.

This must signal a very important event. I presume it is directly ascribable to our success in controlling infectious and nutritional diseases, the triumph of immunization and of antibiotics to control and to cure that category of disease. It speaks about a change in epidemiology; it says that acute diseases of children and young people have been conquered, and they are no longer causes of mortality. Those who in past years died at the age of two from scarlet fever, or at the age of 21 from tuberculosis, or at the age of 14 from polio, no longer die from those causes. They live to a ripe old age. Thus, mortality rates have declined and life spans have increased.

Beyond this change in the prevention of and the capacities to cure the infectious and nutritional diseases, the acute diseases of older adults have become largely cancer, heart and blood vessel diseases, and kidney conditions. The significant aspect of our current epidemiology is the prevalence of chronic diseases, the afflictions of those of us who are called, euphemistically, the golden agers. To put it in the terms that Dr. Lester Evans was so wont to use, "we have succeeded in replacing mortality with morbidity." Death is not the problem so much now as is illness. We must turn our attention from the prevention of death to the handling of illness. To say it in my own words, we now have come to the realization that health service must include two components: one, medical cure of acute disease, and the other, health care which includes the prevention of disease, the care of those whose disease is incurable, and the maintenance of health.

Hunterdon has responded to that dramatic change which occurred almost as it began. To be sure, it built an acute hospital; but its recent building has been an addition of the long-term beds which provide a facility for care, not cure.

It has very substantially enlarged its out-patient facilities, it has created satellite clinics throughout the area; and, lastly, it has built and established special clinics designed to cope with the health problems of alcoholism and drug abuse.

The center has also altered its education program, most importantly by the introduction of the family practice residency as a new venture in medical education designed to meet the needs of health as well as illness. It has also altered its educational concept by realizing that it is not sufficient to be concerned with the education of physicians, nurses, social workers, and health workers of all kinds, but it is also necessary to educate patients as well. This, I think, is a brief description of a process of evolution, geared to the original decisions, concepts, ideas, but adjusting to the necessity of meeting new conditions, new desires, and new wants.

I come now to thinking about the road ahead, the needs of the future, the applicability and the viability of the three ideas I have been concentrating upon—what Hunterdon faces in the next 20 years. One is always on dangerous ground when he begins to gaze into the crystal ball. However, one thing is certain in this world of uncertainty—the future will bring new demands, new needs, new opportunities. Of this I am certain. I will go the next step and say that we can predict with some accuracy some of those demands which the future will bring to this community and to its health facility known as the Hunterdon Medical Center. I expect with confidence that before this century is out, the killer diseases of the middle-aged will be at least understood, and that medical science will be able to do something about them. I expect the process of cancer to yield at least to the point of control, if not of prevention. The processes of hypertension and atherosclerosis will undoubtedly yield to control and perhaps even to prevention. More genetic knowledge and the capacity to apply it and its medical technology will lead to fewer birth defects. More understanding of the mind and the emotions will make some mental diseases at least controllable, if not preventable. Thus, in the future I would predict that the mortality pattern of the middle years of life would be more like that currently of young adults. If I remember my figures correctly, for Americans between the ages of 1 and 39, the greatest cause of mortality is automobile accidents and very close behind that is homicide, including suicide. But the greatest health problem of those years, at least those beyond the teens, is alcoholism and the next problem is drug abuse and certainly high on the list we will have to place obesity. This says that the morbidity pattern—from the age of one day to, say, 59—will show trauma as first, chronic disease as second, and mental disease as third.

Implicit in what I am saying is that the pattern is now clear. With more knowledge we shift from cure after the fact of disease to the control of disease, and with still more knowledge to the prevention of disease. The important point I wish to make is that as this shift of emphasis occurs, the emphasis in health service must shift from healing towards teaching. I would point out to you in the list which I just recited—automobile accidents, homicide, alcoholism, drug abuse, obesity—these are human conditions about which the physician cannot, and in my understanding probably never will, have any silver bullets, effective and incredibly complex operations, or any kind of an immunization. These are health problems which arise from human behavior. Therefore, as I look at that future, the common factor in thinking about our health problems is the responsibility of the patient and the question of how one alters human behavior in a way which would make a positive contribution to his health and therefore to his welfare.

I have now come full circle in my thinking. For, when the Hunterdon Medical Center began, you were concerned about the community, the health of *this* community, the health service needs of this community, and the community's responsibilities therefore. And if there is one thing which one must pick out to describe the success of Hunterdon, it has been the community concern and its community orientation. But I am trying to say now that, more and more in the future, that community participation, that community concern has to be more and more personal, since the future health or the improvement of the health of this community will depend not so much upon group actions as upon personal and individual behavior.

In summary, I will attest to the fact that the three principles which I have chosen to talk about have demonstrated their validity in experience and I would add that they are still valid and they ought to guide you into the future.

Epidemiology will change, and increasing knowledge will change our medical technology. Change will be required and, therefore, the process of evolution at Hunterdon must go on indefinitely. But of the three ideas or concepts the one which seems to be rising now to the position of greatest importance is the concentration upon education. Education of physicians, of course, of primary physicians, of course; but most importantly, of yourselves, your children, and the fellow members of this community.

I suppose the next campaign which the center will run will not be one for dollars, but will be a massive campaign to persuade people to be at least partially responsible for their own health.

AFTERWORD

An anniversary such as the one that we at Hunterdon have just celebrated can be a sobering event. One recalls what were the original goals, one weighs these aspirations against the realities of the present, one looks uneasily into the future.

Stated in the simplest terms, we set out to provide the best medical care possible for our community within the limits of our financial and professional capacities. We assumed without really knowing the parameters of the problem to provide a broad spectrum of medical care for Hunterdon County.

Starting with what, except for our general practitioners, was essentially a clean slate, we were able to innovate as few other communities could. We had extraordinary good fortune in having the early guidance of people like Dr. E. H. L. Corwin, Dr. Lester Evans, and Dr. Clarence de la Chapelle, followed by strong and enlightened professional leadership. In addition, we have enjoyed the most remarkable community support. As a result, it may well be that we have come nearer to providing an organized health care system for Hunterdon County than has any comparable community.

The last 20 years have seen remarkable growth as you will have seen from reading this book. Let me state briefly where we stand today.

The hospital is now 200 beds including 15 psychiatric and 30 intermediate-care beds. Our full-time, hospital-based specialist staff numbers 35, providing most of the specialty services needed, given our size and location.

Three-quarters of the 25 family physicians now practicing in the community received their training at Hunterdon Medical Center. We still need more, but we believe that our present family practice training program will provide them.

To attract the graduates of our program to practice in Hunterdon communities distant from the center, we have opened three family health centers by late 1974 and a fourth should open in 1975. These are essentially offices for groups of up to three family physicians with space provided for the use of social workers, psychologists, visiting nurses, specialists on rotation from the medical center and so forth. Some of these are used as model family practice units for our teaching program. Our board is committed to constructing more such centers if this is necessary to assure the availability of family physicians within reasonable distance of all of our residents.

Income from an endowment fund established by J. Seward Johnson is available to support a patient education and outreach program in two of the family health centers. We will seek funds to extend this service to other low-income areas.

We have a Federally funded comprehensive community mental health unit with 15 in-patient beds providing the services of three full-time psychiatrists, plus the appropriate social workers, psychologists, and therapists. This unit operates a Methadone program and also provides space and a coordinator for a very active voluntary alcoholism program.

A home care program with a full-time nurse director is very active.

The speech and hearing unit carries on an extensive program, cooperating with the school systems.

The pediatric department heads up six programs for handicapped children starting with one providing infant stimulation.

Numerous health-oriented groups such as a prenatal training group, an obesity group, and an emphysema club meet at the center.

We provide space for a county dental program and for

the family nursing service and cooperate with all health-oriented organizations of the county.

Of particular importance, of course, is our commitment to medical education. The major emphasis is on family practice training. Hunterdon was one of the first six hospitals approved by the AMA for its experimental two-year program in 1962. We are now approved for six openings in a three-year program. Last year we had over 100 applicants, all from top American schools, for the six seats.

We are affiliated with the New Jersey College of Medicine and Dentistry-Rutgers Medical School with a commitment to provide training for up to 20 third-year students at all times. We provide openings for a limited number of Rutgers specialty residents on a rotation basis. All of our full-time and a number of our family physicians are on the faculty of the school. Our director is a member of the executive committee of the faculty.

A number of senior students from medical schools in New Jersey and neighboring states pick Hunterdon for their six weeks senior elective.

We provide training for X ray and laboratory technicians and, in cooperation with the local high school, we have an extensive program in practical nurse training.

So much for the present.

We have not fulfilled our expectations in two areas. We tried and failed to establish a pre-paid program for medical care for the entire community. Hopefully, we can accomplish this in the future. In theory, it might be easier under the national health insurance plan. Also, we have not provided adequate long-term nursing home care for low-income and Medicare people. This is our number one priority at present and, hopefully, in cooperation with the county government, we can meet it.

The problems we will face in the future, not only in improving and extending our services but maintaining them, will bring new challenges. The two things that will have the most profound effect on us are the fact that Hunterdon, because of its location, faces an inevitable explosive population growth during the next 20 years and, secondly, that some form of national health insurance seems inevitable in the future.

The growth in the population will be difficult but not impossible to cope with. Our plans as to the expansion of the present building complex, while not specific, are essentially determined. In addition, we own three sites in outlying areas where future satellite hospitals can be built as needed. Our medical school affiliation should assure us of a highly trained specialist staff and our commitment to the family practice residency program and to the construction of family health centers where necessary should assure adequate primary medical coverage.

On the other hand, the effect of the national health insurance program is full of troubling unknowns. Some form of legislation is inevitable. One can do no more than to speculate as to the form such a program will take. The degree of coverage and the resulting governmental controls will increase with time. That seems sure.

There is one problem that any form of national health insurance will create. The public's expectations as to what medical care can and should provide are quite unrealistic. We, as a nation, are convinced that somewhere there exists a silver bullet that can cure any illness and that each of us is entitled to have. We see little reason to take responsibility for our own health if a cure is available. This will be particularly true if the government pays for it. If one applies the concept that absolutely any type of medical care should be available for everyone, not only would the cost be astronomical but the facilities and personnel would, quite simply, be inadequate.

If the only method the government has of controlling costs is to limit the number of dollars available to providers, the stresses and strains in the existing system would increase enormously.

Anne Somers, in her paper, defines three general routes the nation could travel in an effort to solve its health care problems. We are convinced that the only way to create true competition in the health care field is to give organized groups of health care providers comparable per capita allowances, with a mandate to provide total medical care to a given group of people. There is little question in our minds that only in this way can true competition in the health care field exist. We are confident that the Hunterdon Medical Center, organized as it is and working with all the health care agencies in the county, could compete successfully with anyone as to the quality and adequacy of medical care provided and particularly as to patient satisfaction. It is clearly our intention to press ahead, expanding and refining our present system of care.

Thus, as we enter our third decade, we look back with some satisfaction and ahead with some concern. We recognize that we have had extraordinary good fortune in those that have advised and led us and in the community that has supported us so fully. We have indeed been at the right place at the right time. During the next decade new leadership will arise, a new community will come into being and tomorrow's problems will be other than those of today.

Certainly Hunterdon Medical Center has brought a high standard of care to a once inadequately served community. Possibly it has influenced, in a small way at least, the delivery of health care in the nation. Hopefully it will not be overwhelmed by the changes that lie ahead. Our citizens will defend it.

Lloyd B. Wescott
President, Board of Trustees

ABOUT THE CONTRIBUTORS

HIRAM BENJAMIN CURRY, M.D., is Director of the Family
Practice Residency Program at Medical University Hospital, Charleston, South Carolina, and Professor and Chairman of the Department of Family Practice at Medical
University of South Carolina, Charleston. He is medical
director of out-patient clinics at Medical University of South
Carolina, Associate Professor of Neurology at Medical College of South Carolina, and former Chief of Neurology Service at the Veterans Administration Hospital, Charleston. In
1951 he was named a diplomate of the National Board of
Medical Examiners and in 1959 was licensed to the South
Carolina Board of Medical Examiners. Dr. Curry holds a
National Institutes of Health post-doctoral fellowship to
the National Institute of Neurological Diseases and Blindness and received the Outstanding Medical Educator Award
in 1973. He is a consultant to the American Medical Association Residency Review Committee for Family Practice and
a former consultant on family practice to the Surgeon General of the Navy. He presently serves on the South Carolina
Committee on Medical Education, the Task Force on Graduate Medical Education, and the Advisory Council for Improvement of Health Care. Under United States Public
Health Service grants he was principal investigator for a study
on cerebral and cortical blood flow in health and disease and
was co-principal investigator for a study on cardiac and
cerebral vascular sounds. He is the author and co-author of
numerous articles published in medical journals and has delivered several invitational lectures in this country and abroad.

ROBERT R. HENDERSON, M.D., a management consultant in health services, previously was Vice President of Geomet, Inc., of Rockville, Maryland, and before that had been Medical Director of Hunterdon Medical Center from 1960 to 1970. He came to Hunterdon Medical Center in 1953. When he was named medical director of the hospital he was serving as Director of Internal Medicine. Dr. Henderson previously had been chief resident in the chest service section of Bellevue Hospital in New York City. He was for several years staff lecturer in epidemiology and public health at the Yale University School of Medicine and has lectured at Columbia University College of Physicians and Surgeons, the University of Pennsylvania School of Medicine, and other schools. Dr. Henderson has served the United States Public Health Service as consultant and study committee member on a variety of programs including OEO, HUD, Appalachian health programs, and tuberculosis control. He has contributed a number of articles to medical journals and is writing a book on Hunterdon Medical Center and its relationship to national health problems.

FREDERICK J. KNOCKE, M.D., Medical Director of Hunterdon Medical Center since 1971, came to the hospital in 1953 as Director of Orthopaedic Service. He was Associate Medical Director from 1955 to 1971. A graduate of Princeton University, he received his medical degree from Cornell University in 1939. Dr. Knocke was an orthopaedic surgeon with the Third Army in Europe during World War II. He has held teaching affiliations at Columbia and New York Universities and at present is Associate Clinical Professor of Orthopaedic Surgery at the New Jersey College of Medicine and Dentistry-Rutgers Medical School. Dr. Knocke is a fellow of the American Academy of Orthopaedic Surgeons, an executive committeeman and past president of the New Jersey Orthopaedic Society, and a member of the New Jersey Utilization Program and of the Council on Professional Practice of the New Jersey Hospital Association. He and his wife wrote *Orthopaedic Nursing* (Philadelphia: F. A. Davis Co., 1951).

RICHARD M. MAGRAW, M.D., is President of the Norfolk (Va.) Area Medical Center Authority. He was formerly Deputy Executive Dean at the University of Illinois College of Medicine where he was Professor of Internal Medicine and Psychiatry. During a 25-year teaching and administrative association with the University of Minnesota, he took leaves of absence to serve as Assistant Director of Minnesota's Bureau of Health Services for Extramural Relations and as Deputy Assistant Secretary for Health and Manpower in the United States Department of Health, Education, and Welfare. Dr. Magraw is Chairman of the American Medical Association's Advisory Committee on Undergraduate Medical Education and serves on the editorial board of the *Journal of Medical Education*. He has contributed more than 40 articles to professional journals including the *Journal of the American Medical Association, New England Journal of Medicine, American Journal of Psychiatry, Journal-Lancet, Postgraduate Medicine,* and *Annals of Internal Medicine*.

JOHN SCHOFF MILLIS, PH.D., President and Director of the National Fund for Medical Education, is Chancellor Emeritus of Case Western Reserve University and former president of the University of Vermont and of Western Reserve University. His expertise in the field of medical education has been utilized extensively in a wide area of professional service. Dr. Millis currently is a member of the National Board of Medical Examiners and the Educational Council for Foreign Medical Graduates, past chairman of the President's Advisory Panel on Heart Disease, a trustee of the American

Nurses' Foundation, consultant to the American Academy of Orthopaedic Surgeons, and Chairman of the Study Commission on Pharmacy. He has served the educational field and his home community of Cleveland extensively in an advisory and administrative capacity. He holds many honorary degrees from major colleges and universities.

EDMUND D. PELLEGRINO, M.D., is Vice President for Health Affairs and Chancellor of Medical Units at the University of Tennessee and a former director of the Health Sciences Center, State University of New York at Stony Brook. Hunterdon Medical Center's second Medical Director, he held the post from 1955 through 1959 during which time he also was Director of Internal Medicine (1953–1959). He left Hunterdon to become Professor and Chairman, Department of Medicine, University of Kentucky College of Medicine at Lexington. He has served as a consultant to the United States Public Health Service in internal medicine and to the Veterans Administration, Department of Medicine and Surgery, Nursing Service. He has served as Chairman of the Association of American Medical Colleges Planning Committee for the Comparative Study of Teaching Programs in Comprehensive Medicine and has been a member of several committees of the American Medical Association, the American Hospital Association, the National Institute of Health, the United States Public Health Service, and the Association of American Medical Colleges. Dr. Pellegrino is listed in *Who's Who in America*, *Who's Who in the Southeast*, and *American Men of Science*. He is author or co-author of some 100 published articles. He is a diplomate of the National Board of Medical Examiners and of the American Board of Internal Medicine.

ANNE RAMSAY SOMERS, author, lecturer, teacher, and consultant, has been, for the past two decades, involved in studies of health and hospital care and social insurance. She is Associate Professor, Department of Community Medicine, New Jersey College of Medicine and Dentistry-Rutgers Medical School and Research Associate, Industrial Relations Section, Princeton University. Mrs. Somers is a member of the United States Department of Health, Education, and Welfare's Health Insurance Benefits Advisory Council, the American Hospital Association's National Advisory Committee on Health, and the Advisory Committee on Health Services of the Association of American Medical Colleges. She is the author of *Hospital Regulation: The Dilemma of Public Policy* (Princeton: Princeton University Press, 1969) and co-author with her husband, Herman M. Somers, of several additional books. Her articles have appeared in Encyclopaedia Britannica and numerous national medical journals including the *New England Journal of Medicine, Journal of Medical Education, AMA Archives of Environmental Health,* and *Annals of the American Academy of Political and Social Science.* She was co-producer and scriptwriter in 1970 and 1971 for two television films produced by the New Jersey Public Broadcasting Authority— *The Hospital and the Community* and *The Hunterdon Medical Center—One Community's Approach to Comprehensive Health Care.*

RAY E. TRUSSELL, M.D., M.P.H., General Director of Beth Israel Medical Center, New York City, was the first Director of Hunterdon Medical Center, from 1950, three years before the center opened, until 1955. He came to Hunterdon from Albany (N.Y.) Medical College where he was Professor of Preventive Medicine at Columbia University's School of Public Health and Administrative Medicine. On special leave from the university, he held the post of Commissioner of Hospitals of New York City from 1961 to 1965. Dr. Trussell is Professor of Administrative Medicine at Mount Sinai School of Medicine. He is a member of the executive committee of the State Hospital Review and Planning Council of New York State and chaired the council's hospital code committee. He is a fellow of the American Public Health Association. He is a member of the Board of Directors of the Health and Hospital Planning Council of Southern New York and is a former member of the United States Department of Health, Education, and Welfare's Health Insurance Benefits Advisory Council. He is the author of *Hunterdon Medical Center: The Story of One Approach to Rural Medical Care* (Cambridge, Mass.: Harvard University Press, 1956) and, with Dr. Jack Elinson, *Chronic Illness in a Rural Area: The Hunterdon Study* (Cambridge, Mass.: Harvard University Press, 1959).

LLOYD B. WESCOTT, President of the Board of Trustees of Hunterdon Medical Center, started a large dairy farm in Hunterdon County in 1935, an operation that still continues. Over the years he was active in agricultural affairs at the local, state, and national level. As Vice President of the Hunterdon County Board of Agriculture he was asked to chair a committee to study the need for a hospital in the county in 1947. He headed the first fund drive in 1949 and assumed the presidency of the board of the proposed medical center in 1950. This has led to a broad involvement in health care concerns. Mr. Wescott is a member of the executive committee of the National Planning Association and a member of the board of the Prudential Insurance Company. He served for 16 years as Chairman of the Board of Control of the New Jersey Department of Institutions and Agencies. He has received honorary doctorates from Rutgers-The State University and Lafayette College. He is an Honorary Fellow of the American College of Hospital Administrators and is the recipient of the Award of Honor of the American Hospital Association as a member of that organization's Special Committee on the Provision of Health Services.

SAMUEL WOLFE, M.D., M.P.H., DR. P.H., is Director of Community Medicine for Long Island Jewish-Hillside Medical Center, New Hyde Park, New York, and Professor of Community Medicine at the State University of New York at Stony Brook. In the mid-1960s he was Commissioner of the Saskatchewan Medical Care Insurance Commission which implemented the plan which became Canada's universal health insurance program. He also directed lay groups in the development of Canada's first community health centers in Saskatchewan and was consultant to a provincial association of such centers. More recently he was co-director of the Matthew Neighborhood Health Center, the Center for Health Care Research, and the Office of Comprehensive Health Programs at Meharry Medical College in Nashville, Tennessee. Dr. Wolfe is the principal investigator of a long-term study to measure the effects of health care service alternatives. He has published numerous papers and co-authored (with Robin F. Badgley) two books, *Doctors' Strike: Medical Care and Conflict in Saskatchewan* (New York: Atherton, 1967) and *The Family Doctor* (Toronto: Macmillan, 1972).

SELECTIVE BIBLIOGRAPHY

Bambara, A. J. and Hunt, A. D., Jr. "Specialist Plus, Not Versus, Family Physician: A Setting Conducive to Effective Postgraduate Education." *Postgraduate Education,* Vol. 20, No. 3, September 1956.

Cavitch, Barbara. "Parents Assist in Care of Hospitalized Children." *Nursing World,* Vol. 133, No. 5, May 1959.

de la Chapelle, Clarence E. and Jensen, Frode. *A Mission in Action: The Story of the Regional Hospital Plan of New York University.* New York: New York University Press, 1964.

Crane, Almena Dean. "Our Health is Our Wealth." *American Agriculturist,* Vol. 157, No. 20, October 15, 1960.

Elliott, James. "More Ways Than One: A Look at Pluralism in Health Care." *The Lancet,* April 1969.

Furnas, J. C. "We Fetched Ourselves a Medical Center." *Harper's,* June 1952.

Hemmendinger, Miriam. "Rx: Admit Parents at All Times." *Child Study—A Quarterly Journal of Parent Education,* Winter 1956–57.

Henderson, Robert R. "Full-Time Practice in the Community Hospital." *Journal of the American Medical Association,* Vol. 212, No. 12, June 1970.

———— *Hunterdon Medical Center and Its Relationship to National Health Problems.* Work in progress, to be published by Harvard University Press under a grant from the Commonwealth Fund.

"Hospital for the Well." *Architectural Forum,* December 1953.

Hunt, Andrew D., Jr. and Parmet, Morris. "Collaboration Between Pediatrician and Child Psychiatrist in a Rural

Medical Center." *Pediatrics*, Vol. 19, No. 3, March 1957.

Hunt, Andrew D., Jr. and Trussell, Ray E. "They Let Parents Help in Children's Care." *The Modern Hospital*, September 1955.

"A Medical Center Emerges from a Community Survey." *Hospitals*, March 1955.

"Medical Center for the Rural Practitioner." *Journal of the American Medical Association*, Vol. 154, No. 9, February 27, 1954 (advertisement reprinted from *Pfizer Spectrum*).

Medicine in the Changing Order: Report of the New York Academy of Medicine Committee on Medicine and the Changing Order. New York: The Commonwealth Fund, 1947.

Menges, Roger. "Country Doctors Get Medical Center Facilities." *Medical Economics*, March 1953.

"Metamorphosis of a Satellite Health Center." *Group Practice*, April 1971.

Middleton, John. "No Salaried vs. Private Practice Wrangle Here." *Hospital Physician*, November 1968.

Morgan, Mary Louise and Lloyd, Barbara Joyce. "Parents Invited." *Nursing Outlook*, Vol. 3, May 1955.

Parmet, Morris. "The Role of the Full-Time Psychiatrist in the General Hospital." *Journal of the Medical Society of New Jersey*, Vol. 57, October 1960.

Pellegrino, Edmund D. "Role of the Community Hospital in Continuing Education—The Hunterdon Experiment." *Journal of the American Medical Association*, May 25, 1957.

———— "The Role of the Local Community in the Development of Health Services—The Hunterdon Experiment." In *Industry and Tropical Health: IV.* Boston: Harvard School of Public Health, 1961.

Rannels, Herman W. "Obstetrics in a Rural Community." *Postgraduate Medicine*, Vol. 25, No. 2, February 1959.

Somers, Anne Ramsay. "Toward a Rational Community

Health Care System." *Hospital Progress*, Vol. 54, April
1973.

Trussell, Ray E. *Hunterdon Medical Center: The Story of
One Approach to Rural Medical Care.* Cambridge, Mass.:
Harvard University Press, 1956. A Commonwealth Fund
book.

———— and Elinson, Jack. *Chronic Illness in a Rural Area:
The Hunterdon Study.* Cambridge, Mass.: Harvard University Press, 1959.

Tuck, Jay Nelson. "The Family Doctor: Can An Endangered
Species Make a Comeback?" *New York News Magazine*,
August 26, 1973.

Wescott, Lloyd B. "Innovation in Medical Staff Organization." *Hospital Medical Staff*, Vol. 1, No. 3, March 1972.

———— "A Model Medical Center for Comprehensive Care in
the Community." In *Medicine and Society: Contemporary
Medical Problems in Historical Perspective.* Philadelphia:
American Philosophical Society Library, Library Publication No. 4, 1971.

———— "The Role of the Community in Developing Health
Care." *Bulletin of the New York Academy of Medicine*,
2nd series, Vol. 46, No. 12, December 1970.

Wiles, Margaret B. "The Nurse on the Survey Team." *Nursing Outlook*, Vol. 5, No. 2, February 1959.

FILMS

A Matter of Life. Produced and written by Richard Ellison
for WNBC-TV with narration by Chet Huntley. 1967.

The Hunterdon Medical Center—One Community's Approach to Comprehensive Health Care. Co-produced and
written by Anne Ramsay Somers for the New Jersey
Public Broadcasting Authority, 1971.